DASH DIET RECIPES

Easy Dash Diet Recipes for Beginners and Weight Loss

(For Weight Loss and Lower Blood Pressure)

David Fowler

I0092650

Published by Alex Howard

Dash Diet Recipes: Easy Dash Diet Recipes for Beginners and Weight Loss (For Weight Loss and Lower Blood Pressure)

ISBN 978-1-990169-02-1

Legal & Disclaimer

The information contained in this book is not designed to replace or take the place of any form of medicine or professional medical advice. The information in this book has been provided for educational and entertainment purposes only.

Table of contents

Part 1

Introduction

This book contains more recipes based on the Dash Diet. Because the Dash diet was created based on years of research from the National Heart, Lung and Blood Institute studies it is not a passing fad. The initial aim of the diet was to lower high blood pressure without using medication. Along with that another great benefit of the diet is that people also experienced healthy weight loss as a result!

Another benefit of this diet is that there are no extreme measures required to make it work. You can still eat most of the foods that you love.

Weight loss is important not only from a physical point of view but along with obesity comes health problems, like high blood pressure.

For those who already are suffering from high blood pressure and/or are overweight, a diet is advised by doctors. This is where the DASH Diet comes into play. This diet is based on the recommendations for healthy eating from the food pyramid. It outlines more precisely the best options for creating healthy meal plans and maintaining the diet long-term.

Chapter 1: What Is The Dash Diet?

The DASH Diet is designed for one specific purpose, which is outlined in its full name
D: Dietary
A: Approaches to
S: Stop
H: Hypertension
This diet has the secondary benefit of weight loss and other health improvements because it focuses on fruits and vegetables and follows the Food Pyramid's outline for a 2,000 calorie daily intake.
The diet includes whole grains, poultry, fish and nuts so an emphasis on both protein and fiber exists. The importance of extra potassium, magnesium and calcium is also a strong thread to the DASH Diet, so low-fat dairy products are recommended. Limitations are placed on red meats and products that contain high levels of sugar, like sweets and sugary beverages.

A Diet Without Pills or Tricks
The DASH Diet is a reliable diet that is more easily maintained because it focuses on changing your eating habits and pairing that with more exercise. No pills, supplements or tricks are necessary to succeed with this diet. This also makes it easier to maintain, since no additional products need to be purchased.

Instead, it is a healthy way of living that helps you lengthen your life expectancy while losing weight and finding more pleasure in daily life.

Some more benefits to this diet include a reduction in the risk of developing diabetes. A major risk factor for developing diabetes is an unhealthy diet. Another benefit to eating a low- sodium diet you can also reduce the risk of developing osteoporosis.

These and other life-threatening conditions can ultimately reduce your life expectancy if you continue to eat an unhealthy diet. Taking the time to understand how to eat properly can enable you to live a full and healthy life.

Chapter 2: The Dash Diet: Effectiveness

In January of 2014, the DASH Diet was named the best overall diet for lowering weight and blood pressure and for lower cholesterol as well.

According to US News & World Report, the DASH Diet is the best diet overall because of its focus on fruits, vegetables and fish. The plant-based diet is also a high-ranking choice for people following Weight Watchers, since that program does not prohibit eating any specific group of foods.

This is the fourth year in a row the DASH Diet has received best overall diet honors. This shows the longevity of the diet's success. It also shows that people find it works and can be maintained in order to maintain the results that are desired.

Weight Loss

The DASH Diet's main focus is not to lose weight. Instead, it is meant to decrease hypertension. Therefore, the diet is based on 2,000 calories per day, which is what the Daily Food Pyramid already advises. If you can live by this diet for its intended purpose of decreasing hypertension and decrease caloric intake to

1,600 or less per day, the likelihood of losing weight increases drastically.

Part of the problem is that we tend to opt for foods that are quick and easy without really thinking about the nutritional value. As a result our bodies miss out on valuable nutrients that we need to thrive. Over a prolonged period this lack of nutrients can cause serious problems that result in a variety of conditions. This diet helps address the lack of vitamins and minerals in your daily diet. By taking out processed foods and replacing them with fruits and vegetables as well as lean meats it gives our bodies what they need to operate efficiently over the long-term.

Lowering Blood Pressure

The DASH Diet is also helpful because it requires a reduction of the sodium in your diet to less than 2,300 milligrams per day. This helps avoid hypertension, or high blood pressure. If someone who already suffers from hypertension, this diet can help decrease the effects and bring your blood pressure to a more manageable level.

Chapter 3: Using The Dash Diet For Weight Loss

It is important to understand the DASH Diet was not created for weight loss purposes. However, if you begin with the effort to eat healthy and meet the calorie requirements, then aim for a caloric deficit each day (eating less than the recommended daily limit of 2,000 calories), then weight loss can be achieved.

The primary focus of this diet is less fat and sodium while eating a more balanced diet. This is a first step toward weight loss, because you eliminate the foods higher in calories and worse for your system.

The dash diet doesn't really revolve around counting calories. Rather it's about moderation. You can still eat a wide variety of foods that you love as long as you don't overindulge in the foods that can cause problems. Now there are foods that you want to avoid to stay within the guidelines of the dash diet. The list isn't too extensive and there are foods that can be used as replacements.

Sugars

Recently sugar has been implicated in many conditions. In fact sugar has been shown to be pervasive in a lot of the foods that we eat without us really realizing it. A good way to start to understand what products are loaded with sugar is to pay attention to the ingredients on the label. There are many common foods high in sugar which include anything made with white flour and processed, soda and many fruit juices, candy, and white breads and rolls.

Fat

There are many healthy fats that are good for you but others should be limited. Of course trans-fats like those in crackers and some sweet snacks should be avoided. Some oil also should be limited like coconuts and palm oil.

Salt

Because the diet focuses on low sodium that means that you will have to pay attention to which foods are high in sodium and avoid them. The aim is to reduce your salt intake to a healthy level without overdoing other ingredients that can cause health problems. Some typical foods which are high in sodium include potato chips, soy sauce, can or processed meats, canned foods like spaghetti and chilli as well as can beans or other vegetables.

When you look at it this is actually a pretty short list compared to all of the choices in the supermarket. Focus on all the great things that this diet encourages that will improve your health and energy.

Chapter 4: Your Weekly Diet Plan

Making a daily plan for the DASH Diet means meeting the recommendations for a certain number of servings of different food types.

The recommendation follows:

· **Whole grains (6 to 8 servings a day)**

· **Vegetables (4 to 5 servings a day)**

· **Fruits (4 to 5 servings a day)**

· **Low-fat or fat-free milk and milk products (2 to 3 servings a day)**

· **Lean meats, poultry and fish (6 or fewer servings a day)**

· **Nuts, seeds and beans (4 to 5 servings a week)**

· **Fats and oils (2 to 3 servings a day)**

· **Sweets, preferably low-fat or fat-free (5 or fewer a week)**

· **Sodium (no more than 2,300 mg a day)**

Following these guidelines means a six-week plan must stay consistent, yet it must contain variety so you are likely to stay interested and not go off-diet.

Serving sizes:

Grains:

· 1 slice bread
· 1 oz dry cereal
· ½ cup cooked rice, pasta, or cereal

· ½ small bagel

Vegetables

· 1 cup raw leafy vegetables (about the size of a baseball)
· ½ cup raw or cooked vegetables
· 4 oz vegetable juice

Fruits

· 4 oz fruit juice
· 1 medium fruit
· ¼ cup dried fruit
· ½ cup fresh, frozen, or canned fruit

Milk Products

· 8 oz milk
· 1 cup yogurt
· 1 ½ oz cheese

Meats, Poultry, and Fish

· 3 oz cooked lean meats, poultry, or fish

Nuts, Seeds, and Dry Beans

· 1/3 cup or 1 ½ oz nuts
· 2 Tbsp or ½ oz seeds
· ½ cup cooked dry beans or peas

Fats and Oils

- 1 tsp soft margarine
- 1 Tbsp lowfat mayonnaise
- 2 Tbsp light salad dressing
- 1 tsp vegetable oil

Sweets

- 1 Tbsp sugar
- 1 Tbsp jelly
- ½ oz jelly beans
- 8 oz lemonade

Chapter 5: Dash Diet Transition

Transitioning to the dash diet is relatively straightforward because some of the benefits include having more energy as well as feeling better in general. However if you are moving from a diet with sugary carbs you may temporarily have a few digestive changes. Because fresh fruits and vegetables have a lot more fiber there may be some changes which are temporary in nature. This is totally natural and it's just your body getting rid of some of the toxins in your system. This will likely only last or a week or two. This is just a minor inconvenience when you look at the overall benefits of this healthy diet.

Slow changes

Now the first week will probably be more about lowering your sodium intake while increasing the amount of fresh fruit and vegetables. It will also include phasing out sugary white bread and pastries. If you switch to whole-grain bread it will help lessen some of the side effects of switching to this higher fiber diet.

Exercise

Exercise is a strong step toward combatting health issues and the stigmas that come with being overweight.

However, exercise must be paired with a healthy diet in order to reach optimal success. There are the recommendations from the Food and Drug

Administration via the food pyramid. These advise a 2,000 calorie daily diet and include certain servings from each of four food groups. This is helpful.

Chapter 6: Recipes

Breakfast

Recipe: English Muffin Breakfast Sandwich

· ½ whole-wheat, English muffin
· 1 slice reduced-fat Swiss cheese, in pieces to fit muffin
· Olive oil
· ½ cup liquid egg substitute, seasoned
· 1½ tsp. scallion, finely chopped (green part only)

1.   Toast the muffin in an oven toaster or broiler. Turn off the toaster.
2.   With the cheese pieces, top the muffin and for about 30 seconds, let stand until the cheese is melted by the residual heat and then transfer to plate.
3.   Spray a small non-stick skillet with the oil and heat over medium heat and then add the egg substitute and for about 15 seconds, cook until the edges are set. Lift the edges of the egg substitute using a heatproof spatula so the uncooked liquid can flow underneath.
4.   Continue with cooking and every 15 seconds, lift the edges until egg mixture is set, about 1½ in total. Fold the edges of the egg mixture into the center to make a rough-shaped "patty" about 3 inches across using the spatula.

5. Sprinkle with the scallion after transferring the egg patty to the muffin. Serve hot.

Recipe: Cream Cheese And Strawberry Topped Tartine

· 1 slice bread, whole-grain
· 2 tbsp. spreadable fat-free cream cheese
· 2 large, hulled and sliced strawberries
· 1 tsp. honey (optional)

1. Toast the bread using a toaster.
2. Spread the cream cheese first then top with the strawberries.
3. You may drizzle with the honey, if available.
3.

Recipe: Omelette Topped With Pepper Jack Cheese And Broccoli

· Olive oil
· ½ cup liquid egg substitute, seasoned
· 1 slice reduced-fat pepper Jack cheese, torned into pieces
· ¼ cup broccoli, warmed in a microwave, cooked and chopped

1. Using the Olive oil, spray a small non-stick skillet then heat over medium heat. Put the egg substitute and for about 15 seconds, cook until edges are set.
2. Lift the edges of the egg substitute using a heatproof spatula so the uncooked liquid can flow

underneath. As you continue cooking, lift the edges every 15seconds until the omelette is set for about 1½ minutes in total.

3.   Remove from the heat then, scatter the cheese and broccoli over the top of the omelette. Use the spatula to help the omelette fold over on itself into thirds while tilting the pan slightly.

4.   Slide to a plate then serve.

Recipe: Healthy Granola

· ¼ cup light brown sugar, packed
· 2 tbsp. water
· 1 tbsp. vegetable oil
· 1 tsp. ground cinnamon
· 1 tsp. maple flavoring or vanilla extract
· 4 cups old-fashioned oats, rolled
· 1 cup dark raisins
· ½ cup dates, chopped
· ½ cup milk, fat-free, for serving
·

1.   At 300°F, preheat the oven.

2.   Whisk together the brown sugar, water, oil, cinnamon, and maple flavoring in a large bowl until the sugar is dissolved then add the oats and mix until it is lightly coated. Spread evenly on a large rimmed baking sheet.

3. Stirring occasionally and bringing the toasted edges in toward the center of the granola, Bake until the oats are evenly crisp for about 40 minutes. Stir in the raisins and dates after removing from the oven and let it cool completely. For about 2 weeks, store in an airtight container.

4. For each serving, scoop ½ cup of granola into a bowl and add milk.

4.

Recipe: Oatmeal With Spice And Apple

· 1 sweet apple, cored and peeled, cut into ½-inch dice
· ⅔ cup water
· ⅓ cup old-fashioned oats, rolled
· Pinch of ground cinnamon
· Pinch of nutmeg, freshly grated
· A few grains of kosher salt
· ½ cup milk, fat-free, for serving
·

1.   Combine the apple, water, oats, cinnamon, nutmeg, and salt in a small saucepan. Bring to a boil, from medium heat then reduce the heat to low and then cover. For about 4 minutes, simmer until the oats are tender.
2.   To microwave: Combine the apple, water, oats, cinnamon, nutmeg, and salt in a 1-quart microwave-safe bowl. Cover with plastic wrap tightly and on high power, microwave until the oats are tender for about 4 minutes. Stir, and let stand for 1 minute after you uncover carefully.
3.   Transfer the oatmeal and pour in the milk to a bowl and serve.
3.

Recipe: French Toast With Cinnamon-Almond And Raspberry Sauce

Raspberry Sauce
· 2 (6 oz.) containers fresh raspberries (about 2⅔cups), or 1 (12-ounce) bag thawed frozen raspberries
· 1 tbsp. amber agave nectar
· 2 tsp. lemon juice, fresh

French Toast
· 1 large egg
· 1 large egg white
· ½ tsp. ground cinnamon
· ¾ cup milk, 1% low-fat
· 1 tbsp. amber agave nectar
· ½ tsp. vanilla extract
· ¼ tsp. almond extract
· Canola oil
· 8 slices whole-wheat (or multigrain) bread
· ½ cup natural almonds, toasted and sliced, for serving
· 1 (6 oz.) container fresh raspberries (about 1⅓ cups), for serving (optional)
·

To make the sauce:
1.   Until the berries are smooth, pulse the raspberries, agave, and lemon juice in a food processor or blender.

(Don't puree too much to prevent raspberries seed from crushing giving it a bitter taste)

2.   To remove the seeds, strain through a fine-meshed wire strainer. Then, set aside at room temperature.

To make the French toast:

1.   At 200°F, preheat the oven.

2.   Whisk together the egg and egg white in a large, wide bowl and whisk in the cinnamon until it is well distributed. Afterwards, whisk in the milk, agave, vanilla, and almond extract also.

3.   Heat over medium heat after spray a large griddle or non-stick skillet with oil. Dip a bread slice into the egg mixture to moisten, but not soak, the bread in batches. Reduce the heat to medium-low as you place on the griddle. For about 2 minutes, cook until the underside is browned.

4.   With a wide spatula, flip the French toast and cook until the other side is browned for about 2 minutes more thcn, transfer to a baking sheet and while cooking the remaining French toast, keep warm in the oven.

5.   Place 2 slices of French toast on a plate for each serving topped with 3 tablespoons of the sauce and then sprinkle with 2 tablespoons of almonds. If desired, you may add a few fresh raspberries then serve immediately.

Recipe: Pancakes With Maple-Strawberry Compote

Compote
· 1 pound (fresh) strawberries, hulled and coarsely chopped
· ¼ cup maple syrup
Pancakes
· 1 cup pastry flour, whole-wheat
· ½ cup all-purpose flour, unbleached
· 1 tbsp. sugar
· 1½ tsp. baking powder
· ¼ tsp. kosher salt
· 1½ cups milk, 1% low-fat
· 1 large egg
· 2 large egg whites
· 2 tbsp. canola or corn oil

To make the compote:
1.   In a medium bowl, mix the strawberries and maple syrup.
2.   At room temperature, let stand to allow the strawberries to release their juices for at least 1 hour and up to 4 hours.

To make the pancakes:
1.   At 200°F, preheat the oven.

2.   In a medium bowl, mix the baking powder, flour (unbleached), pastry flour (whole-wheat), sugar, and salt. Whisk together the egg and egg whites, milk, and the 2 tablespoons oil then pour into the dry ingredients and stir until just combined in another bowl.

3.   Over medium-high heat, heat a non-stick griddle and spray with the oil. For each pancake, pour ¼ cup of the batter onto the griddle. For about 2 minutes, cook until the top surface of each pancake is covered with bubbles,.

4.   With a wide spatula, flip the pancakes and for about 1 minute longer, continue cooking until the undersides are golden brown.

5.   While making the remaining pancakes, transfer the pancakes to a baking sheet and keep warm in the oven. Topped with the compote, serve the pancakes hot.

Lunch

Recipe: Sirloin Rubbed With Curry Plus Peanut Sauce Dipping

Sirloin

· 1 tsp. curry powder
· ½ tsp. ground ginger
· ½ tsp. garlic, granulated
· ½ tsp. kosher salt
· ½ tsp. black pepper, freshly ground
· Canola oil in a spray pump
· 1¾ pounds of 1 in. thick sirloin steak (excess fat trimmed)

Peanut Dipping Sauce

· ¼ cup peanut butter, smooth
· 3 tbsp. cold black tea, brewed
· 3 tbsp. coconut milk, light
· 2 tsp. fresh ginger, peeled and minced
· 2 tsp. soy sauce, reduced-sodium
· 1½ tsp. rice vinegar
· 2 tsp. curry powder
· 1 clove garlic, crushed
· Fresh cilantro, chopped, for garnish

To prepare the sirloin:

1. In a small bowl, mix the salt and pepper, curry powder, ground ginger, garlic.

2.   Spray the oil on both sides of the steak and season with the curry mixture.

3.   Let stand at room temperature while making the peanut sauce.

To make the Peanut Dipping Sauce:

1.   Whisk together the tea, peanut butter, ginger, coconut milk, soy sauce, vinegar, curry, and garlic in a medium bowl,.

2.   At about 4 inches, position a broiler rack from the source of heat and preheat on high. Put oil in the broiler rack and add the steak.

3.   Flip the steak over after 3 minutes then broil until browned on both sides and until the meat feels only slightly resilient when center-pressed, for about 6 minutes for medium-rare.

4.   Let it stand for 3 minutes after transferring to a carving board.

Recipe: Stir-Fried Sirloin, Shiitake, And Asparagus

Sauce
· ¾ cup canned low-sodium chicken broth
· 2 tbsp. dry sherry (or dry vermouth)
· 1 tbsp. rice vinegar
· 1 tbsp. soy sauce, low-sodium
· 1 tbsp. corn starch
· ½ tsp. black pepper, freshly ground

Stir-Fry
· 4 tsp. canola oil
· 1 pound sirloin steak (excess fat trimmed), cut across the grain into ¼-inch-thick slices and then into 2-inch strips
· 1 tbsp. fresh ginger, peeled and minced
· 2 cloves minced garlic
· 12 oz. thin asparagus (woody stems discarded) cut into 1-inch lengths
· 6 oz. sliced shiitake mushroom caps
· 6 oz. trimmed sugar snap or snow peas
· ½ cup water
· 3 (1 inch length-cut) scallions, white and green parts

To make the sauce:
1.   In a small bowl, whisk together the broth, sherry, vinegar, corn-starch, and pepper, soy sauce.
To make the stir-fry:

1.   In a large non-stick skillet, heat over medium-high 2 teaspoons of the oil.
2.   Add the steak in two batches and stirring occasionally, cook until seared for about 2 minutes.
3.   Transfer to a plate then heat the remaining 2 teaspoons oil in the skillet over medium-high heat. For about 30 seconds, add the ginger and garlic and stir until fragrant.
4.   Mix in the asparagus, shiitake, and sugar snap peas and stir well. While stirring, add the water and cook until the water has evaporated and the vegetables are crisp- tender for about 3 minutes.
5.   Stir in the scallions during the last minute. Add the sauce mixture to the skillet and stir for about 30 seconds until thickened and boiling.
6.   Return the steak to the skillet and stir well and transfer to a serving platter.
7.   Serve while hot.
7.

Recipe: Beef-Mushroom Mixed With Sour Cream–Dill Sauce

·

2 tsp. canola oil
· 1 pound sirloin steak (excess fat trimmed) cut across the grain in ½-inch-thick slices and then into 2-inch-wide pieces
· 12 oz. sliced cremini mushrooms
· ¼ cup shallots, finely chopped
· 2 tsp. cornstarch
· ¾ cup Homemade Beef Stock
· ½ cup sour cream, reduced-fat
· 1 tbsp. fresh dill, finely chopped
· ½ tsp. kosher salt
· ½ tsp. black pepper, freshly ground

1.   Spray a large non-stick skillet with oil and heat over medium-high heat.
2.   Put in half of the sirloin and cook while flipping the sirloin pieces halfway through cooking, until browned on both sides for about 2 minutes then transfer to a plate. Do the same with the remaining sirloin.
3.   Over medium heat, heat the 2 teaspoons oil in the skillet. Stirring occasionally add the mushrooms and cook until their liquid evaporates and they begin to brown for about 6 minutes. Stir in the shallots and for about 1 minute cook until softened.
4.   Sprinkle the corn-starch over the broth and stir to dissolve in a small bowl. Stir into the mushrooms and

continue cooking until boiling and thickened. Mix in the dill, sour cream, salt and pepper.

5.   To the skillet, return the sirloin and any juices on the plate and for about 30 seconds, cook just until heated through.

6.   Serve hot.

Recipe: Filet Mignon With Bourbon-Shallot Sauce

· 1 tbsp. four-peppercorn blend
· 4 (6-oz.) filets mignons
· 1 tsp. canola oil
· ¼ cup shallots, finely chopped
· ¼ cup Cognac, bourbon, brandy
· 1 cup Homemade Beef Stock
· 1 tbsp. cold butter, unsalted
· Pinch of kosher salt

1.   Under a heavy skillet, coarsely crush the peppercorns in a mortar and pestle or on a work surface.

2.   Combine the 1 teaspoon oil and the shallots in the skillet and cook over medium heat while stirring until the shallots soften for about 2 minutes. Add the bourbon and for about 1 minute, cook until almost completely evaporated. Add the stock and bring to a boil over high heat, with a wooden spatula, scraping up the browned bits in the skillet.

3. For about 2 minutes, boil until reduced to a half cup. Remove from the heat and whisk in the butter and salt.

4. Serve each steak topped with a spoonful of sauce on a dinner plate.

4.

Recipe: Roast Spiced Eye Of Round

· 1 tsp. cumin seeds
· 1 tsp. coriander seeds
· ½ tsp. black peppercorns, whole
· ½ tsp. kosher salt
· ½ tsp. ground ginger
· ¼ tsp. black pepper, freshly ground
· ⅛ tsp. cayenne pepper
· 1 (3-lbs.) tied beef eye of round roast
· 1 clove garlic (cut into about 12 slivers)
· Olive oil

1.   In the center of the oven, position a rack and at 400°F, preheat the oven.
2.   Coarsely crush together the coriander, cumin, and peppercorns in a mortar, in an electric spice grinder, or on a work counter under a heavy skillet. Transfer to a bowl and add the salt, ginger, pepper, and cayenne.
3.   Make 1-inch-deep incisions in the beef using the tip of a small knife, and stuff garlic clove sliver into each slit. Spray the beef with oil and sprinkle with the spice mixture.
4.   On a meat rack, place the roast in a roasting pan then roast for 10 minutes. At about 350°F, reduce the oven temperature and continue roasting until the instant- read thermometer inserted in the beef reads 125°F for medium-rare for about 1 hour.
5.   Let stand for 10 minutes after transferring the beef to a carving board. Remove the string and cut the meat

into thin slices crosswise. Transfer to a serving platter and pour the carving juices over the beef.

6.   Serve immediately.

Recipe: Peppered Beef Fajitas

· 2 tsp. olive oil
· 1 pound cut across the grain in half inch thick slices sirloin steak (excess fat trimmed) and then into 2-inch-wide pieces
· 1 cored and cut into ¼-inch-wide strips large red bell pepper
· 1 cored and cut into ¼-inch-wide strips large green bell pepper
· 1 thin half-moon-cut medium red onion
· 2 minced cloves garlic,
· 1 tbsp. Mexican Seasoning
· 12 (8-in.) flour tortillas, for serving
· Lime wedges, for serving

1.   Heat over medium-high heat a large non-stick oil-sprayed skillet. Add half of the sirloin and cook, flipping the sirloin pieces halfway through cooking, until browned on both sides for about 2 minutes. Transfer to a plate. Do the same with the remaining sirloin.
2.   Heat the 2 teaspoons oil in the skillet over medium-high heat. Add the bell peppers, garlic, and onions. Cook while stirring occasionally until tender for about 7 minutes. Stir in the beef with any juices and the Mexican Seasoning and transfer to a platter.
3.   Fill a flour tortilla or lettuce leaf with the beef mixture and squeeze lime juice on top to serve.
4.   Rollup and serve.
4.

Recipe: Ground Sirloin With Pinto Chili

· 1 tbsp. olive oil
· 1 chopped medium yellow onion
· 1 cored and chopped medium green bell pepper
· 2 minced cloves garlic
· 1¼ pounds ground sirloin
· 2 tbsp. chili powder
· ½ tsp. pure ground chipotle chili,
· cayenne (optional)
· ½ tsp. kosher salt
· 1 (28-oz.) can undrained reduced-sodium chopped tomatoes in juice,
· 2 (15-oz.) cans drained and well rinsed reduced-sodium pinto beans,

1.   Over medium heat, heat the oil in a large saucepan. Add the onion and bell pepper and for about 3 minutes, cook while stirring occasionally until softened. Stir in the garlic and cook for about a minute until fragrant.

2.   Add the sirloin and cook, stirring often and breaking up the meat with the side of the spoon for about 6 minutes until it loses its raw look. Stir in the chili powder and salt, and cook for 1 minute, stirring often.

3.   Stir in the tomatoes with their juice and bring to a boil over high heat. Return the heat to medium and cook at a brisk simmer while stirring occasionally until the juices have thickened slightly for about 15 minutes.

4. Add the beans and cook for about 5 minutes until heated through. If you prefer a thicker chili, mash some of the beans into the cooking liquid using a large spoon. Spoon into bowls.

5. Serve hot.

5.

Dinner

Recipe: Roast Beef Salad

· 4 medium beets (1 pound), scrubbed (unpeeled)
· 2 tbsp. cider vinegar
· 1½ tbsp. pared and freshly grated horseradish
· 2 tbsp. olive oil
· 1 large cored and cut into ½-inch dice Rome apple,
· 1 finely chopped scallion (white and green parts)
· 12 oz. thinly sliced Roast Spiced Eye of Round

1. Preheat the oven to 400°F.
2. In aluminum foil, wrap each beet and place on a rimmed baking sheet. Bake until beets are tender (pierce with tip of a small knife to check) for about 1¼ hours.
3. Unwrap and let cool then, peel the beets and cut into ½-inch dice.
4. Whisk together the horseradish and vinegar in a medium bowl, then whisk in the oil. Add the scallion apple and beets and mix thoroughly. For at least 1 hour or up to 1 day, cover and refrigerate until chilled,
5. Among four dinner plates, divide the beet salad and top with equal amounts of the sliced roast beef.
6. Serve chilled.
6.

Recipe: Spinach With Strawberry Salad

· 1 pound hulled fresh strawberries
· 2 tbsp. balsamic vinegar
· 2 tbsp. olive oil, preferably extra-virgin
· 2 tbsp. water
· Pinch of kosher salt
· Pinch of freshly ground black pepper
· 2 tsp. poppy seeds
· 7½ cups (6 oz.) baby spinach
· ½ cup hazelnuts, skinned, toasted, and chopped coarsely
· 4 oz. (1 cup) crumbled goat cheese (optional)
·

1.   Chop coarsely ¼ cup of the strawberries and transfer to a blender. Slice the other strawberries and set aside.
2.   Puree the vinegar, water, chopped strawberries, oil, salt, and pepper until smooth in the blender. Pulse once or twice as you add the poppy seeds just to combine.
3.   In a large bowl, toss the baby spinach and strawberry dressing. Afterwards, add the hazelnuts and reserved sliced strawberries and toss again. Sprinkle with the goat cheese, if available.
4.   Serve at once.
4.

Recipe: Bulgur And Beef Meat Loaf

· 1 cup boiling water
· ½ cup bulgur
· 2 tsp. canola oil
· 1 chopped medium yellow onion
· 1 cored and cut into ¼-inch dice medium red bell pepper,
· 2 minced cloves garlic
· ¼ cup plus 2 tbsp. low-salt tomato ketchup
· 1 tbsp. Worcestershire sauce
· 1 tsp. kosher salt
· ½ tsp. black pepper, freshly ground
· 2 large egg whites
· 1 pound ground sirloin

1.   Combine the boiling water and bulgur in a heatproof medium bowl and let stand until the bulgur has softened and absorbed the water for about 20 minutes.
2.   Preheat the oven to 350°F. Line a rimmed baking sheet with aluminum foil and spray with oil.
3.   Over medium heat, heat the 2 teaspoons oil in a medium non-stick skillet. Add the bell pepper, onion and garlic and cook until tender while stirring occasionally for about 6 minutes. Transfer to a bowl and cool slightly.
4.   Drain the bulgur in a wire sieve, pressing hard on the bulgur to extract the excess water. Add to the bowl with the vegetables, and then stir in ¼ cup of the

ketchup, salt, and pepper and Worcestershire sauce. (adding the ingredients at this point prevents egg whites from being cooked) Stir in the egg whites. Add the ground sirloin and mix just until combined. Shape into an 8 × 4-inch loaf on the foil-lined baking sheet.

5.   For about 40 minutes, bake until the loaf is golden brown and an instant-read thermometer inserted in the center reads 165°F.

6.   Spread the top of the loaf with the 2 tablespoons ketchup during the last 5 minutes.

Recipe: Pork Chop Topped With Mustard Sauce

· Canola oil
· 6 (4-oz.) ½ inch thick boneless pork loin chops
· ½ tsp. kosher salt
· ½ tsp. freshly ground black pepper
· 2 tsp. corn starch
· ½ cup canned low-sodium chicken broth
· ½ cup milk, 1% low-fat
· 1 tbsp. Dijon mustard
· 1 tbsp. butter, unsalted
· 2 tbsp. shallots, minced
· 2 tsp. fresh tarragon, chopped

1.   Heat over medium heat a large oil-sprayed non-stick skillet. Add to the skillet the seasoned salt and pepper-seasoned pork.
2.   For about 3 minutes, cook until the undersides are golden brown. Flip the pork and cook for about 3 minutes more until the other sides are golden brown and the meat feels firm when pressed in the thickest part with a fingertip. Transfer to plate.
3.   In a small bowl, whisk the corn starch into the broth. Add the mustard and milk and whisk again; set aside for a while.
4.   Over medium heat, melt the butter in the skillet. Add the shallots and cook while stirring often until tender for about 2 minutes. Whisk the broth mixture, pour into the skillet, and bring to a boil. Return the pork with any juices on the plate to the skillet and cook

while turning occasionally for about 1 minute up until the sauce thickens.

5.   Cut each chop in half after transferring the pork to a deep platter. Pour the sauce over the pork chops and sprinkle with the tarragon.

6.   Serve hot.

6.

Recipe: Pork Chops And Cabbage

Red Cabbage
· 1 slice of coarsely chopped reduced-sodium bacon
· 1 tsp. canola oil
· 1 chopped medium yellow onion
· 1 small cored and thinly sliced red cabbage (1¼ pounds),
· ¼ cup cider vinegar
· 2 cored and cut into ½-inch dice Granny Smith apples
· ¼ cup water
· 3 tbsp. grade B maple syrup
· ¼ tsp. kosher salt
· ¼ tsp. black pepper, freshly ground

Pork Chops
· Canola oil
· 4 (4-oz.) boneless center-cut pork chops (excess fat trimmed)
· ¼ tsp. kosher salt
· ¼ tsp. black pepper, freshly ground

To prepare the red cabbage:
1.   Cook the bacon in the oil, stirring occasionally in a medium saucepan over medium heat until the bacon is crisp and brown for about 5 minutes.
2.   Add the onion and cook while stirring occasionally up until golden for about 5 minutes. Stir in the cabbage in three or four additions, sprinkling each addition with a tablespoon or so of the vinegar.

3.   Stir in the water, salt and pepper, maple syrup, apples. Reduce the heat to medium-low and cover tightly. Cook while stirring occasionally until the cabbage is very tender for about 1 hour. Add a couple of tablespoons of water if the liquid cooks away.

To prepare the pork:

1.   Heat over medium heat a large non-stick oil-prayed skillet

2.   Season the pork with the salt and pepper and add to the skillet. Cook until the undersides are golden brown for about 3 minutes. Flip the pork and cook until the other sides are golden brown and the meat feels firm when pressed with a fingertip in the thickest part for about 3 minutes more.

3.   Transfer to a plate and tent with foil to keep warm.

Recipe: Pork Chops With Rosemary And Balsamic Glaze

· Olive oil
· 4 (4-oz.) ½ inch thick boneless pork loin chops
· 1 tbsp. fresh rosemary, finely chopped
· ½ tsp. kosher salt
· ½ tsp. black pepper, freshly ground
· ¼ cup balsamic vinegar

1.   Heat over medium heat a large oil-sprayed skillet.
2.   Season the pork with the salt, pepper, and rosemary. Add to the skillet and cook until the undersides are golden brown for about 3 minutes.
3.   Flip the pork and cook while adjusting the heat as needed so the pork cooks steadily without burning up until the other sides are browned and the pork feels firm when pressed in the center with a fingertip for about 3 minutes more. Transfer the chops to a dinner plate.
4.   Add the vinegar to the skillet, off heat. (Do not inhale the strong fumes) Scrape up the browned bits in the bottom of the skillet using a wooden spoon. The heat of the skillet should be enough to evaporate the vinegar to about 2 tablespoons. Return the skillet to medium heat to reduce the vinegar slightly if necessary.
5.   Over each chop, drizzle the glaze

6. Serve hot.

6.

Recipe: Pork Tenderloin With Bbq Sauce

· 1½ pounds pork tenderloin, trimmed excess fat
· 1 tsp. kosher salt
· ½ tsp. freshly ground black pepper
· 1 tbsp. canola oil
· 2 tbsp. all-fruit peach spread
· 2 tbsp. no-salt-added tomato ketchup
· 1 tbsp. cider vinegar
· 1 tsp. chili powder
· ½ tsp. hickory liquid smoke flavoring (optional)

1. Preheat the oven to 350°F.
2. Season the pork with salt and pepper. Tie down the folded thin ends of the tenderloin with kitchen twine so the meat is thickened evenly. With an ovenproof handle over medium heat, Heat the oil in a large non-stick skillet. Add the tenderloin and cook while turning occasionally up until it is browned on all sides for about 5 minutes.
3. Mix the chili powder, peach spread, vinegar, ketchup, and liquid smoke (if using) in a small bowl. Spread over the tenderloin and then, transfer the skillet with the tenderloin to the oven and bake until an instant-read thermometer inserted in the tenderloin reads 145°F for about 12 to 15 minutes.
4. Let stand for 5 minutes after transferring the pork to a carving board. Remove the strings and cut the tenderloin crosswise into ½-inch-thick slices. Arrange

on dinner plates and pour any carving juices on top. Serve while hot.

4.

Dessert

Recipe: Banana-Berry Smoothie

- ½ ripe banana, preferably frozen
- ½ cup fresh or frozen blueberries
- ½ cup low-fat (1/%) milk
- ½ cup plain low-fat yogurt
- ¼ teaspoon vanilla extract
- 1 tablespoon amber agave nectar (optional)

1. Peel and cut the banana into chunks.
2. Puree the ingredients including the sweetener, if available, in blender until smooth.
3. Pour into a tall glass
4. Serve immediately.

Recipe: Peanut Butter And Choco Smoothie

- · 1 ripe banana (frozen overnight)
- · ⅔ cup milk, 1% low-fat
- · ⅔ cup plain yogurt, low-fat
- · 2 tbsp. peanut butter, chunky
- · 2 tbsp. cocoa powder, unsweetened
- · 1 tbsp. amber agave nectar (if available)
- · 4 ice cubes

1. Peel the banana and cut it into chunks.
2. Puree the banana with the milk, yogurt, peanut butter, cocoa powder, sweetener (if available), and ice cubes in a blender.
3. Pour into two tall glasses
4. Serve immediately.

Recipe: Borecole And Apple Smoothie

· 1 cup stemmed and loosely packed kale leaves, well washed
· ½ sweet apple, such as Jonathan or Gala, cored and coarsely chopped
· ⅓ cup apple cider
· 2 tablespoons sunflower seeds
· 6 ice cubes
· 8 fresh mint leaves
·

1. In a blender, puree all ingredients until smooth.
2. Pour into a tall glass
3. Serve immediately.

Recipe: Mango-Flavored Lassi

· 1 ripe pitted, peeled, and coarsely chopped mango
· ½ cup plain yogurt, non-fat
· ½ cup milk, fat-free
· 3 ice cubes
· Pinch of ground cardamom (optional)
·

1.   Puree the mango, yogurt, milk, and ice cubes in a blender until smooth.
2.   Pour into a tall glass. If available, sprinkle with the cardamom.
3.   Serve immediately.

Recipe: Coconut-Papaya Shake

· 1 ripe seeded, peeled papaya, and cut into 1-inch chunks
· 1 cup plain yogurt, low-fat
· 1 cup coconut water (different from coconut milk)
· 2 tbsp. wheat germ
· ½ tsp. sweetener, zero-calorie (optional)
·

1.   Including the sweetener (if available), puree all ingredients in a blender.
2.   Pour into two tall glasses.
   3.   Serve.

Recipe: Cranberry-Walnut-Stuffed Baked Apples

· 4 baking apples, such as Braeburn or Rome
   · ½ lemon
· ⅓ cup dried cranberries
· ⅓ cup walnuts, chopped
· 6 tbsp. grade B maple syrup
· ¼ tsp. ground cinnamon
· ¼ tsp. freshly grated nutmeg
· 4 tsp. unsalted butter
· 1 cup boiling water

1. At 350°F, preheat the oven.
2. Cut off the top inch of an apple to make a "lid" one at a time. Scoop out the core with a melon baller, stopping about ½ inch from the bottom of the apple. Remove the top half of the apple skin using a vegetable peeler. With the lemon half, rub the exposed flesh all over.
3. Mix the walnuts, cranberries, 2 tablespoons of the maple syrup, nutmeg and cinnamon in a medium bowl. Stuff the apples with the mixture and then top each with 1 teaspoon of butter. Replace the apple "lids."
4. Transfer to a baking dish that is large enough to hold the apples. Over the apples, squeeze the lemon juice from the lemon half. Pour in the boiling water and cover tightly with aluminium foil and bake for 20

minutes. Uncover and baste with the liquid in the baking dish. Continue baking until the apples are tender when pierced with the tip of a small, sharp knife for about 20 to 30 minutes more, depending on the size of the apples. Let stand for 5 minutes after removing from the oven.

5.   Each with 1 tablespoon maple syrup, transfer each apple to a dessert bowl and drizzle.

6.   Serve warm

Recipe: Fresh Berry-Sprinkled Buttermilk Panna Cotta

· 3 tsp. gelatin powder, unflavored
· ¼ cup plus 2 tbsp. low-fat (1%) milk
· 2¾ cups buttermilk
· ½ cup amber agave nectar or honey
· ½ tsp. vanilla extract
· Canola oil
· ½ cup fresh blueberries
· ½ cup fresh raspberries

1.   Sprinkle the gelatin over the milk in a small heatproof bowl and let stand for about 5 minutes until the gelatin absorbs the milk. Add enough water to a small skillet to come ½ inch up the sides and bring to a simmer over low heat. Put the bowl with the gelatin in the water and with a small heatproof spatula, stir constantly for about 2 minutes until the gelatin is melted and completely dissolved.

2. In a medium saucepan, over medium-low heat, warm the buttermilk while stirring constantly, until it is warm to the touch. To prevent curdling, do not overheat. Afterwards, remove from the heat. Add in the gelatin mixture and whisk until combined then whisk in the agave and vanilla. Transfer to a pitcher or a large measuring cup.

3. Oil six 6-oz. ramekins. Pour mixture into the ramekins equal amounts of the buttermilk. Cover each with plastic wrap. For at least 4 hours up to 2 days, refrigerate until chilled and set.

4. Run a dinner knife around the inside of each ramekin, making sure to reach the bottom to break the air seal. Place a plate over the top of the ramekin working with one panna cotta at a time. Give them a firm shake to unmold the panna cotta holding the ramekin and plate together, onto the plate. If stubborn, dip the ramekin (right side up) in a bowl of hot water and hold for 10 seconds, dry, invert and try unmolding again.

Dash Diet Recipes In 15 Minutes

Tomato Basil Omelet

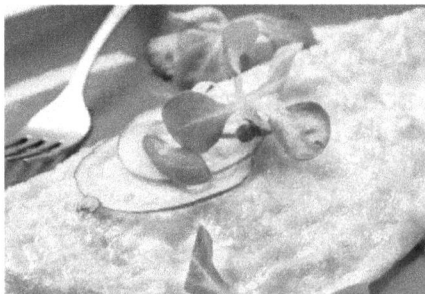

Servings: 1

Ingredients:
- 2 teaspoons olive oil
- 1 medium vine-ripened tomato, chopped
- ¼ cup diced yellow onion
- 1 clove minced garlic
- 2 large eggs, beaten well
- Salt and pepper to taste
- 1 to 2 tablespoons fresh chopped basil

Instructions:
1. Heat 1 teaspoon oil in a small skillet over medium heat.
2. Add the tomato, onion and garlic – sauté for 2 to 3 minutes until tender.
3. Spoon the vegetables off into a bowl and reheat the skillet with the remaining oil.
4. Beat the eggs then pour them into the skillet and season with salt and pepper.
5. Cook for 2 to 3 minutes until the eggs start to set on the bottom.
6. Spoon the vegetables over half the omelet and sprinkle with fresh basil.
7. Fold the egg over the filling then cook for another 1 to 2 minutes until the egg is set.

Chocolate Raspberry Smoothie

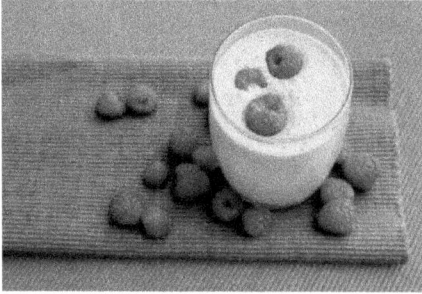

Servings: 1

Ingredients:
- 1 ½ cups frozen raspberries
- 1 cup fat-free milk
- ½ cup nonfat Greek yogurt, plain
- 2 tablespoons unsweetened cocoa powder
- 1 to 2 packets powdered stevia
- ¼ teaspoon vanilla extract

Instructions:
1. Combine all of the ingredients in a high-speed blender.
2. Pulse the ingredients several times to combine.
3. Blend on high speed for 30 to 60 seconds until smooth and well combined.
4. Pour the smoothie into a glass and enjoy immediately.

Ham And Cheddar Egg Muffins

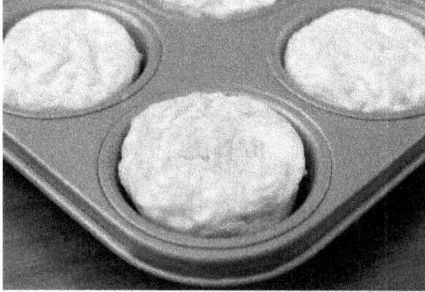

Servings: 12

Ingredients:
- 12 large eggs, beaten well
- ½ cup non-fat milk
- ½ cup diced ham, low-sodium
- 1 green onion, sliced thin
- Salt and pepper to taste
- 1 cup reduced-fat shredded cheddar cheese

Instructions:
1. Preheat the oven to 350°F and grease a 24-cup mini muffin pan with cooking spray.
2. Beat together the eggs and milk in a mixing bowl until light and fluffy.
3. Add the ham and green onion then season with salt and pepper to taste.

4. Stir well then spoon the mixture into the prepared pan.
5. Sprinkle the cheese evenly over the muffin cups.
6. Bake for about 15 minutes or so until the eggs are set – cool for 5 minutes before serving.

Avocado Walnut Lime Smoothie

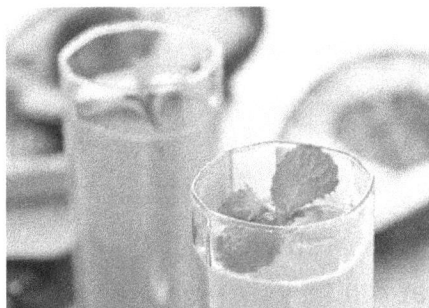

Servings: 1

Ingredients:
- 1 small frozen banana, peeled and sliced
- ½ small ripe avocado, pitted and chopped
- 1 cup fat-free milk
- ½ cup ice cubes
- ¼ cup chopped walnuts, raw
- 2 tablespoons fresh lime juice
- 1 teaspoon raw honey

Instructions:

1. Combine all of the ingredients in a high-speed blender.
2. Pulse the ingredients several times to combine.
3. Blend on high speed for 30 to 60 seconds until smooth and well combined.
4. Pour the smoothie into a glass and enjoy immediately.

Instant Cinnamon Raisin Oatmeal

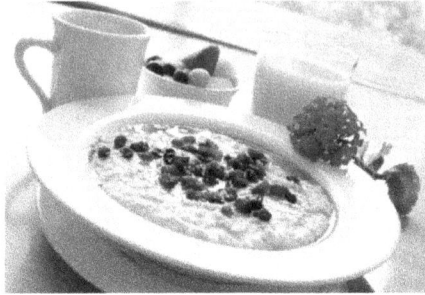

Servings: 1

Ingredients:
- 1 cup nonfat milk
- ½ cup rolled oats, uncooked
- ½ teaspoon ground cinnamon
- Pinch of salt
- ¼ cup seedless raisins
- 1 to 2 teaspoons raw honey

Instructions:
1. Stir together the milk, oats, cinnamon and salt in a microwave-safe bowl.
2. Heat on high for 3 minutes or until thick.
3. Stir well then top with raisins and drizzle with honey to serve.

Mushroom Onion Scramble

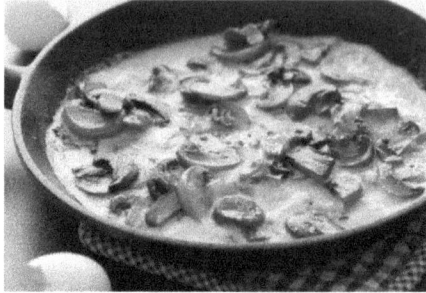

Servings: 4

Ingredients:

- 2 teaspoons olive oil
- 1 ½ cups sliced crimini mushrooms
- ½ cup diced yellow onion
- 2 cloves minced garlic
- Salt and pepper to taste
- 6 large eggs, beaten well
- 2 tablespoons fat-free milk
- 1 to 2 tablespoons fresh chopped parsley

Instructions:

1. Heat the oil in a medium skillet over medium-high heat.
2. Add the mushrooms, onion and garlic then season with salt and pepper.

3. Cook the mixture, stirring often, for 5 to 6 minutes until the vegetables are tender.
4. Beat the eggs with the milk in a small bowl and season with salt and pepper.
5. Pour the eggs into the skillet and cook for another 5 to 6 minutes until the eggs are done to the desired temperature.
6. Sprinkle with fresh chopped parsley to serve.

Warm Vegetable Quinoa Salad

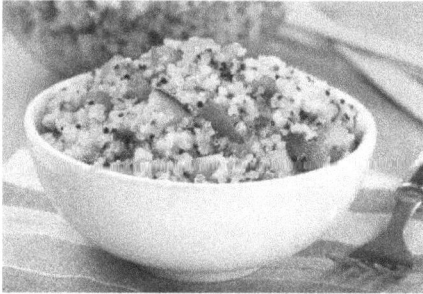

Servings:

Ingredients:
- 2 cups water
- 1 cup uncooked quinoa, rinsed and drained
- 1 tablespoon olive oil
- ½ medium zucchini, diced

- ½ small red pepper, cored and diced
- ½ small yellow pepper, cored and diced
- ½ small red onion, diced
- 1 clove minced garlic
- 1 tablespoon fresh lemon juice
- 1 tablespoon fresh chopped parsley
- Salt and pepper to taste.

Instructions:

1. Whisk together the water and quinoa in a microwave-safe bowl.
2. Heat on high heat for 5 minutes until the quinoa has absorbed the water – fluff with a fork and set aside.
3. Heat the oil in a medium skillet over medium heat.
4. Add the zucchini, bell peppers, onion and garlic – sauté for 5 to 6 minutes until tender.
5. Stir in the cooked quinoa along with the lemon juice and parsley.
6. Season with salt and pepper to taste and serve warm.

Greek-Style Turkey Wrap

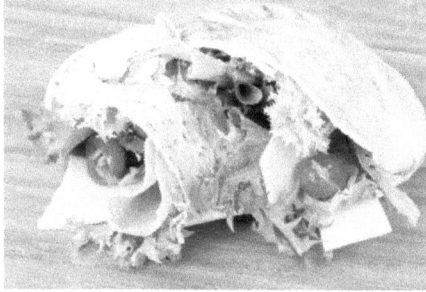

Servings: 1

Ingredients:
- 1 whole-wheat pita
- 2 tablespoons hummus (your choice of flavors)
- 4 thin slices low-sodium turkey breast
- 1 cup chopped green leaf lettuce
- ½ small green pepper, sliced thin
- ½ cup cherry tomatoes, halved
- 2 tablespoons sliced black olives
- 2 tablespoons crumbled low-fat feta cheese

Instructions:
1. Cut the pita in half and open up each half into a pocket.
2. Spread 1 tablespoon of hummus along the bottom of each half.
3. Divide the turkey, lettuce, peppers and tomatoes between the two halves.

4. Add 1 tablespoon of sliced black olives to each half along with 1 tablespoon each of crumbled feta cheese then serve.

Chilled Avocado Soup

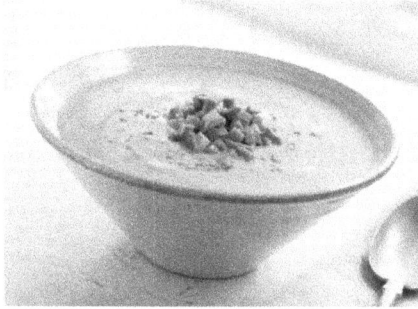

Servings: 6

Ingredients:

- 4 medium ripe avocadoes, halved and pitted
- 1 ½ cups water
- 2 ½ cups fat-free milk
- ½ cup raw cashew halves
- ½ cup diced red onion
- 1/3 cup fresh chopped dill
- 1 ½ tablespoons white wine vinegar
- 1 teaspoon salt

Instructions:

1. Spoon the avocado flesh into a food processor.
2. Add the milk, water, cashews, and red onion then blend to combine.

3. Blend in the fresh dill along with the vinegar and salt.
4. Pour the soup into a bowl then cover and chill for at least 1 hour before serving.
5. Serve cold garnished with mince avocado and a pinch of paprika.

Chicken Apple Pecan Salad

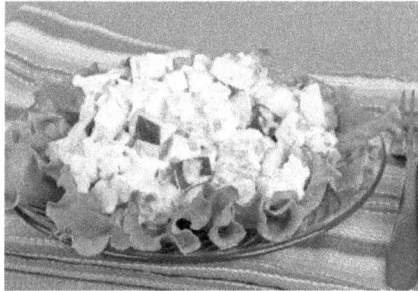

Servings: 8 to 10

Ingredients:
- ½ cup fat-free Greek yogurt, plain
- ½ cup reduced-fat mayonnaise
- 2 to 3 tablespoons fresh lemon juice
- 1 lbs. boneless skinless chicken breast, cooked and chopped
- 2 medium ripe apples, cored and diced
- 2 large stalks celery, diced

- 1 cup chopped pecans

Instructions:

1. In a mixing bowl, whisk together the yogurt, mayonnaise, and lemon juice.
2. Toss in the chicken, apples, celery, and pecans.
3. Serve chilled over a bed of lettuce or on whole-wheat bread.

Kale And White Bean Soup

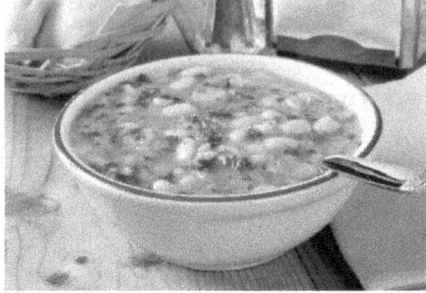

Servings: 4 to 6

Ingredients:
- 1 teaspoon olive oil
- 1 ½ cups chopped yellow onion
- 1 tablespoon fresh minced garlic
- 4 cups low-sodium chicken broth
- 2 (15-ounce) cans white cannellini beans, rinsed and drained
- 4 to 6 cups fresh chopped kale
- Salt and pepper to taste

Instructions:
1. Heat the oil in a large saucepan over medium-high heat.
2. Add the onion and garlic then sauté for 4 to 5 minutes until tender.

3. Pour the broth into a microwave-safe bowl and eat on high for 3 minutes.
4. Add the drained beans to the saucepan then pour in the broth.
5. Bring to a boil then gently mash the beans with a potato masher.
6. Add the kale then season with salt and pepper to taste.
7. Simmer for 4 to 6 minutes on medium heat until heated through. Serve hot.

Balsamic Spinach Avocado Salad

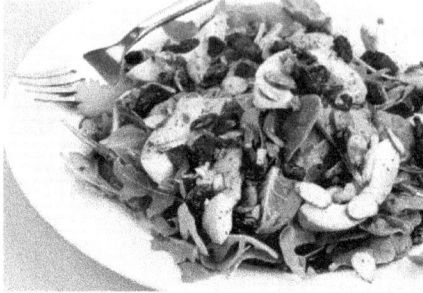

Servings: 4

Ingredients:
- 6 to 8 cups fresh chopped spinach
- 1 medium ripe avocado, pitted and sliced
- ¾ cups seedless raisins
- ½ cup thinly sliced almonds
- ¼ cup olive oil
- ¼ cup balsamic vinegar
- 1 teaspoon raw honey
- ½ teaspoon Dijon mustard
- Pinch garlic powder

Instructions:
1. Toss together the spinach, avocado, raisins and almonds.
2. Divide the mixture between four salad plates.

3. Whisk together the remaining ingredients in a small bowl.
4. Drizzle the dressing over the salads and serve with fresh cracked pepper.

Easy Tomato Basil Soup

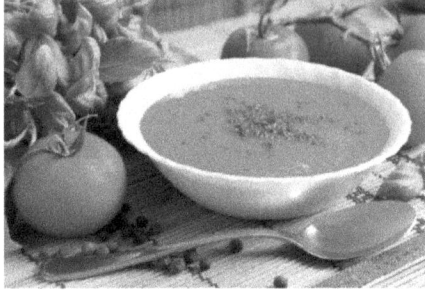

Servings: 4 to 6

Ingredients:
- 1 teaspoon olive oil
- 2 small yellow onions, diced
- 1 tablespoon fresh minced garlic
- Salt and pepper to taste
- 1 (28-ounce) can crushed tomatoes
- 4 cups low-sodium chicken broth
- ½ cup half-n-half
- ¼ cup fresh chopped basil

Instructions:
1. Heat the oil in a large saucepan over medium heat.
2. Add the onions and garlic then season with salt and pepper to taste.
3. Sauté for 3 to 4 minutes until the onions are tender.

4. Stir in the tomatoes and chicken broth then season with salt and pepper again.
5. Bring to a boil then reduce heat and simmer for 10 minutes.
6. Remove from heat and puree the soup using an immersion blender.
7. Whisk in the half-and-half and basil then simmer, if needed, until heated through.

Bbq Chicken Quesadilla

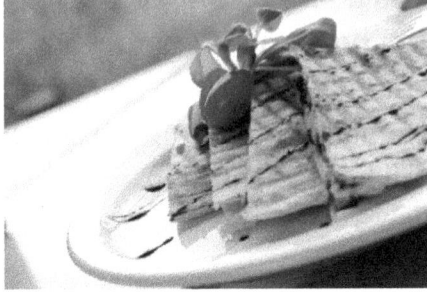

Servings: 1

Ingredients:
- 2 6-inch whole-wheat tortillas
- 1 tablespoon fat-free sour cream
- 1 tablespoon barbecue sauce
- ½ cup shredded chicken breast
- ¼ cup reduced-fat shredded Mexican cheese
- 2 tablespoons diced red onion

Instructions:
1. Lay one of the tortillas out flat.
2. Stir together the sour cream and barbecue sauce then spread on the tortilla.
3. Top with chicken, cheese, and red onion.
4. Place the other tortilla on top then transfer to a greased skillet that has been preheated over medium-high heat.

5. Cook the quesadilla for 1 minute then flip and cook for another minute.
6. Slide the quesadilla onto a plate then cut into quarters to serve.

Cucumber Red Onion Dill Salad

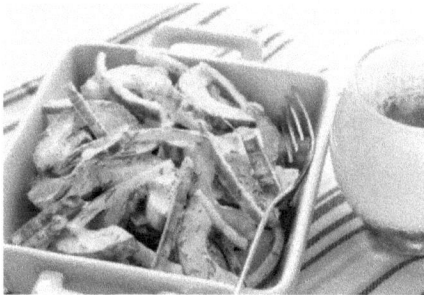

Servings: 4 to 6

Ingredients:
- 2 large English cucumbers, sliced thin
- 1 tablespoon salt
- 2 tablespoons olive oil mayonnaise
- 1 ½ tablespoons white wine vinegar
- 1 teaspoon white sugar
- 2 tablespoons fresh chopped dill
- 1 medium red onion, sliced thin

Instructions:

1. Place the cucumber in a colander and sprinkle with salt.
2. Let drain for 10 minutes then rinsed well with cold water and press to remove as much moisture as possible.
3. In a mixing bowl, whisk together the mayonnaise, vinegar, sugar and dill.
4. Toss in the cucumbers and red onion then serve immediately.

Chicken Tortilla Soup

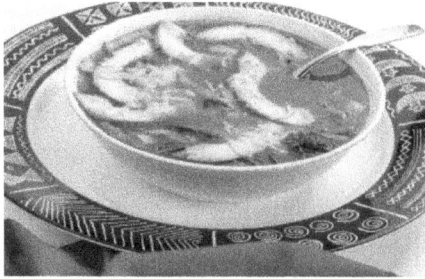

Servings: 8 to 10

Ingredients:
- 1 tablespoon olive oil
- 1 medium yellow onion, chopped
- 1 jalapeno, seeded and minced
- 1 tablespoon fresh minced garlic
- 4 cups low-sodium chicken broth
- 1 (28-ounce) can crushed tomatoes
- 1 (15-ounce) can black beans or red kidney beans, rinsed and drained
- 2 cups rotisserie chicken, shredded
- 1 cup frozen corn
- 1 tablespoon chili powder
- 2 teaspoons fresh lime juice
- 1 ½ teaspoons ground cumin
- ¼ teaspoon cayenne

- Salt and pepper to taste
- 1 ripe avocado, pitted and sliced thin
- 1 cup reduced-fat shredded cheddar cheese

Instructions:

1. Heat the oil in a large stockpot over medium-high heat.
2. Add the onion, jalapeno and garlic – sauté for 3 to 4 minutes until just tender.
3. Stir in the chicken broth, tomatoes, beans, chicken, and corn.
4. Add the chili powder, lime juice, cumin, and cayenne then season with salt and pepper to taste.
5. Bring to a boil then reduce heat and simmer on medium for 5 minutes.
6. Stir in the cilantro and boil for 1 minute more and then adjust seasonings to taste.
7. Spoon into bowls and top with sliced avocado and cheddar cheese to serve.

Black Bean Cheddar Wrap

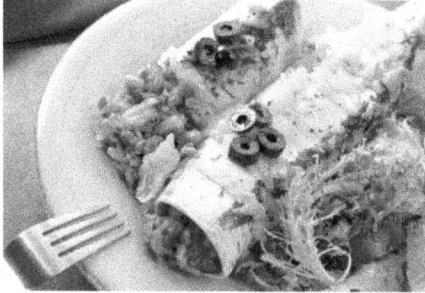

Servings: 1

Ingredients:

- ¼ cup canned black beans, rinsed and drained
- 1 8-inch whole-wheat tortilla
- 2 tablespoons reduced-fat cheddar cheese
- ¼ teaspoon ground cumin
- Pinch of paprika

Instructions:

1. Place the beans in a bowl and mash them gently with a fork.
2. Lay the tortilla out flat and spoon the beans down the middle.
3. Sprinkle with cheddar cheese, cumin and paprika.
4. Roll up the tortilla and microwave on high for 30 seconds until hot.

5. Serve with sliced black olives and tomato salsa, if desired.

Coconut Crusted Tilapia Fillets

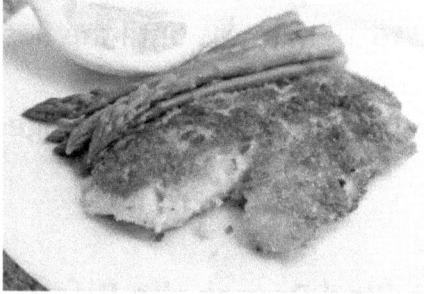

Servings:

Ingredients:
- 4 (4 to 6-ounce) boneless tilapia fillets
- Salt and pepper to taste
- ½ cup unsweetened shredded coconut
- ½ cup whole-wheat breadcrumbs, plain
- ½ teaspoon garlic powder
- 1 large egg, beaten
- Lemon wedges

Instructions:
1. Preheat the oven to 375°F and line a baking sheet with foil.
2. Season the fillets with salt and pepper to taste.
3. Combine the coconut, bread crumbs and garlic powder in a shallow dish.

4. Beat the egg in another shallow dish then dip the fillets in it.
5. Coat the fillets in the coconut mixture and place them on the baking sheet.
6. Bake for 12 to 15 minutes until the flesh flakes easily with a fork.
7. Serve the fillets hot with lemon wedges.

Grilled Portobello Burgers

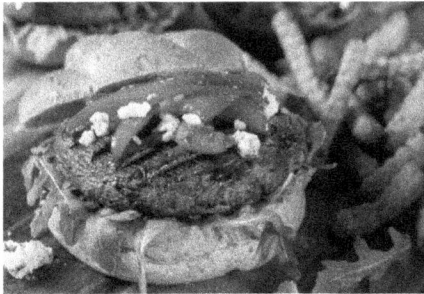

Servings: 1

Ingredients:
- 1 large Portobello mushroom cap, stem removed
- 1 tablespoon olive oil
- 2 teaspoons balsamic vinegar
- 1 clove minced garlic
- 1 whole-wheat bun, toasted

Instructions:

1. Preheat a grill pan over medium-high heat and spray with cooking spray.
2. Place the mushroom cap in a shallow bowl or dish.
3. Whisk together the oil, balsamic vinegar, and garlic then pour over the mushroom cap.
4. Turn the mushroom cap to coat then grill for 3 to 4 minutes on each side until tender.
5. Serve the mushroom cap on a toasted whole-wheat bun with your favorite burger toppings.

Creamy Pesto Parmesan Pasta

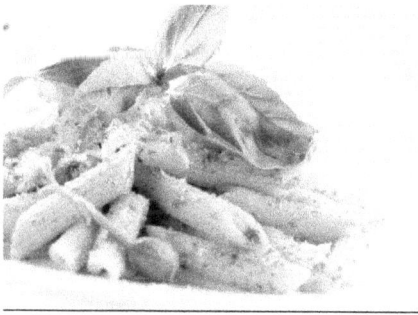

Servings: 4 to 6

Ingredients:

- 10 ounces whole-wheat penne pasta

- 1 teaspoon olive oil
- ½ small yellow onion, diced
- 2 cloves minced garlic
- ½ cup basil pesto
- ¼ cup freshly grated reduced-fat parmesan cheese

Instructions:

1. Bring a large pot of salted water to boil.
2. Add the pasta and cook to al dente according to the directions, about 8 to 10 minutes.
3. Meanwhile, heat the olive oil in a large skillet over medium heat.
4. Add the onion and garlic then sauté until the pasta is done.
5. Drain the pasta then stir it into the skillet along with the pesto and parmesan cheese.
6. Cook for 1 to 2 minutes until heated through then serve hot.

Grilled Balsamic Salmon Fillets

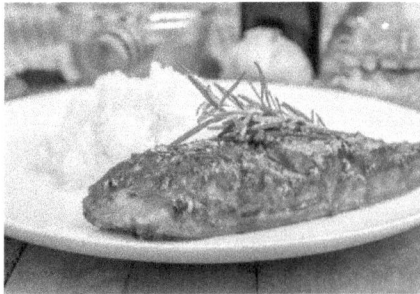

Servings: 4

Ingredients:

- 4 (4 to 6-ounce) boneless salmon fillets
- Salt and pepper to taste
- ¼ cup fresh lemon juice
- 2 tablespoons olive oil
- 1 ½ tablespoons balsamic vinegar
- ¼ teaspoon garlic powder

Instructions:

1. Season the fillets with salt and pepper to taste then place them in a shallow dish.
2. Whisk together the remaining ingredients and pour over the salmon, turning to coat.
3. Let the salmon soak for 15 to 30 minutes.
4. Preheat the grill to medium-high heat and brush the grates with oil.
5. Place the fillets on the grill and cook for 3 to 4 minutes on each side until opaque.

Cinnamon Baked Bananas

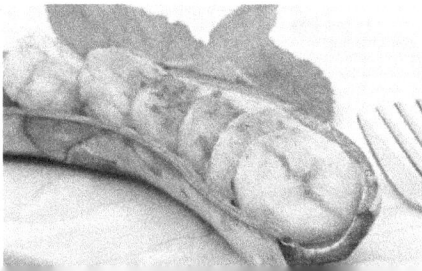

Servings: 6 to 8

Ingredients:
- 1 cup water
- 1/3 cup raw honey
- 1 tablespoon cornstarch
- 2 tablespoons coconut oil
- 2 teaspoons fresh lemon juice
- ½ teaspoon ground cinnamon
- Pinch salt
- 6 to 8 ripe bananas, peeled and sliced

Instructions:
1. Preheat the oven to 350°F and lightly grease a square glass baking dish with cooking spray.
2. Whisk together the water, honey and cornstarch in a small saucepan.
3. Bring to a boil then remove from heat and whisk in the coconut oil, lemon juice, cinnamon and salt.
4. Spread the sliced bananas in the baking dish then drizzle with the sauce.
5. Bake for 10 to 15 minutes until the bananas are tender. Serve hot.

Chocolate Chia Seed Pudding

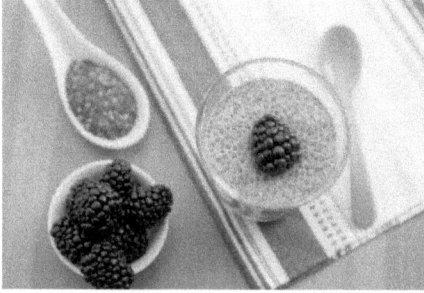

Servings: 4

Ingredients:
- 1 ½ cups fat-free milk
- ¼ cup chia seeds
- ¼ cup unsweetened cocoa powder
- 6 to 8 pitted Medjool dates
- ½ teaspoon vanilla extract

Instructions:
1. Combine all of the pudding ingredients in a high-speed blender.
2. Blend on high speed for 1 to 2 minutes until thoroughly combined.
3. Spoon the pudding into dessert cups.
4. Serve immediately or chill for 1 to 2 hours before serving.

Quick Cinnamon Peach Crisp

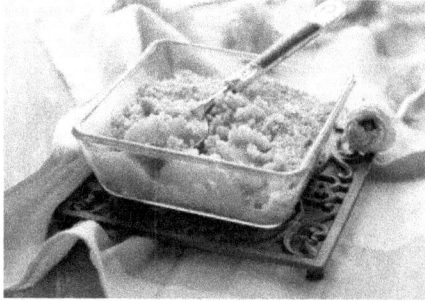

Servings: 4

Ingredients:

- ½ to 1 cup whole-grain granola
- 2 tablespoons coconut oil
- 4 large ripe peaches, peeled, pitted and sliced
- 2 tablespoons raw honey
- ½ teaspoon ground cinnamon

Instructions:

1. Preheat the broiler in your oven to high heat.
2. Spread out the granola on a rimmed baking sheet and broil for 1 to 2 minutes until toasted.
3. Heat the coconut oil in a large skillet over medium heat
4. Stir in the peaches and cook for 2 to 3 minutes.

5. Add the honey and cinnamon then cook 1 minute more until the honey is melted.
6. Divide the peach mixture among four dessert cups and sprinkle with toasted granola to serve.

Microwave Baked Apple

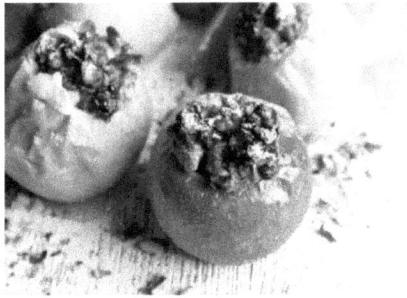

Servings: 1

Ingredients:
- 1 medium ripe apple
- 1 tablespoon seedless raisins
- 1 teaspoon chopped pecans
- 1 teaspoon raw honey
- 1 teaspoon coconut oil, melted
- Pinch ground cinnamon
- ½ cup water

Instructions:

1. Use a small, sharp knife to remove the core from the apple, leaving the bottom intact.
2. Peel the top of the apple about ½-inch down from the stem.
3. Place the apple in a microwave-safe bowl.
4. In another bowl, stir together the raisins, pecans, honey, coconut oil, and cinnamon.
5. Spoon the mixture into the apple then pour the water into the bowl around it.
6. Cover the bowl with plastic wrap, leaving a small gap to vent steam.
7. Microwave on high heat for 5 minutes or until the apple is tender.
8. Transfer the apple to a small plate to serve.

Conclusion

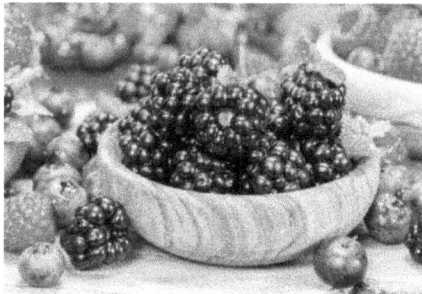

As you have already learned, the DASH Diet was developed as a dietary alternative to blood pressure medication for hypertensive adults. The diet is not intended to be a fad diet – it is founded on sound nutritional principles to help you improve your eating habits and to boost your nutrition. In improving your nutritious you can work to lower your high blood pressure and improve your health overall. The best part is that you don't have to count calories or restrict yourself! The DASH Diet is easy to follow, especially with this book of 15-minute recipes. If you are curious to try the DASH Diet for yourself, then simply pick a recipe from this book and get cooking!

Part 2

Introduction

Dietary Approaches to Stop Hypertension or what is popularly known as Dash Diet was developed in the 1990s for the sole purpose of finding a healthy means to lower one's blood pressure. This diet includes the consumption of more fruits and vegetables, nuts, low fat dairy, and lean meat.

The Dash Diet is effective in lowering blood pressure and in promoting weight loss because the food served are mostly rich in calcium, magnesium, potassium, and fiber; and one that has low salt content. Having all these nutrients present in your diet correct the balance of electrolyte in your body and help in excreting extra fluids that cause high blood pressure. This diet is also effective in weight loss because said nutrients are usually lacking in overweight people, so the Dash Diet can help a great deal in correcting said deficiencies.

This book is filled with Dash Diet recipes that you can easily follow. The dishes are mostly consist of fruits and vegetables, lean meat, and with just a pinch of salt added to food. So flip through the pages and get started with your Dash diet journey to a healthier and leaner you!

Thanks again for downloading this book, I hope you enjoy it!

Chapter 1 – Dash Diet Breakfast Recipes

Recipe #1 - Egg Salad On Cucumber Disks

For the egg salad
- 2 pieces eggs, hardboiled, halved lengthwise, separate yolks from whites
- Dash of Spanish paprika
- ½ tsp. mayonnaise
- Pinch of sea salt
- Pinch of white pepper, to taste

For the cucumber disks
- 4 pieces cucumber disks, about ¼-inch thick, sliced diagonally
- 1 Tbsp. apple cider vinegar
- Pinch of salt
- Pinch of black pepper

Directions:

1. For the egg salad, put together egg yolks, Spanish paprika, mayonnaise, salt, and white pepper in a small bowl. Adjust seasoning if needed. Place inside the fridge to chill for 1 hour or until ready to use.
2. For the cucumber disks, combine cucumber disks, apple cider vinegar, salt, and black pepper in a small bowl. Drain immediately so the cucumbers won't lose their crispness.
3. To serve, layer cucumber disks on a plate. Scoop equal amounts of the egg salad into the hollowed out, egg whites. Serve immediately.

Recipe #2 - Plantain With Egg And Kale

Ingredients:
- 2 pieces eggs, soft-boiled
- 1 plantain, almost-ripe, quartered
- ½ pound fresh kale, roughly chopped with the tough stems removed
- ½ tsp. olive oil
- Pinch sea salt
- Pinch of black pepper, to taste

Directions:

1. Pour olive oil into a non-stick skillet.
2. Fry quartered plantains for 3 minutes or until golden brown. Turn down the heat to the lowest setting.
3. Stir in kale leaves. Stir well. Secure the lid and allow the kale leaves to cook for 2 minutes. Turn off the heat. Season with salt and pepper.
4. To serve, put desired amount of plantain hash into a plate. Serve with soft boiled egg and kale on the side.

Recipe #3 - Warm Oats With Avocado (Beverage)

Ingredients:
- 1 cup water
- ¼ cup steel-cut oats
- ½ ripe avocado, pitted
- ½ cup almond milk
- 1 tsp. stevia

Directions:

1.Pour water and oats into a saucepan. Allow the mixture to boil. Reduce the heat to lowest setting. Cook oats for 25 minutes, stirring often.

2.Remove from the heat. Let the oats cool before transferring into the blender.

3.Add in avocado, almond milk, and stevia. Blend beverage until a smooth and creamy consistency is achieved.

4.Pour desired amount of beverage into cups. Serve.

Recipe #4 - Spinach Pancakes With Tonkatsu Sauce

Ingredients:
- 1 egg
- 1 cup flour
- 3/4 cup water
- 1/4 teaspoon salt
- 1 tsp. olive oil, add more if needed
- 2 cups fresh spinach leaves, chopped
- Tonkatsu sauce, store-bought

Directions:

1.Combine egg, flour, water, and salt in a bowl. Mix well until all ingredients are well-combined.

2.Meanwhile, heat the olive oil in a nonstick skillet. Pour batter and mix in the spinach leaves. Cook for 2 minutes or until set. Flip on the other side and cook for another minute.

3.Repeat the same cooking procedure until the rest of the batter is used up.

Recipe #5 - Coconut Congee

Ingredients:
- ¼ cup tapioca pearls
- 2 cans coconut cream, divided
- 6 cups water
- ¼ cup ripe jackfruit, shredded
- 1 can whole corn kernels
- ¼ cup brown rice
- ⅛ cup palm sugar, crumbled
- pinch of sea salt
- 1 banana, sliced thinly

Directions:

1. Combine tapioca pearls and 1 can of coconut cream in a saucepan. Pour water, water, jackfruit, corn kernels, brown rice, palm sugar, and salt. Stir mixture well Secure the lid and cook for 20 minutes.

2. Pour the remaining can of coconut cream. Adjust seasoning if needed.

3. To serve, ladle congee into bowls. Garnish with banana slices. Cool slightly before serving.

Recipe #6 - Arroz A La Cubana

Ingredients:
For the filling
- 1 white onion, minced
- 1 garlic clove, minced
- ¼ cup lean ground beef
- ¼ cup lean ground pork
- ½ cup frozen peas, thawed
- 1½ Tbsp. Worcestershire sauce
- 1½ Tbsp. tomato puree
- 1½ Tbsp. tomato sauce
- ¼ cup raisins
- 1 bird's eye chili, minced
- ½ Tbsp. sea salt
- Pinch of black pepper, to taste

- 4 eggs
- 3 plantain, ripe, halved lengthwise
- 1½ cups brown rice, cooked
- Pinch of sea salt, to taste
- Olive oil, for greasing

Directions:

1. For the filling, pour a small amount of olive oil into a nonstick skillet. Saute onion and garlic for 3 minutes or until limp and translucent.

2. Stir in lean ground pork and beef. Stir-fry for 2 minutes. Add in peas, Worcestershire sauce, tomato

puree, tomato sauce, raisins, bird's eye chili, salt, and pepper.

3.Reduce the heat to lowest setting. Cook filling for 15 minutes. Adjust seasoning if needed.

4.For the eggs, pour small amount of olive oil. Cook eggs sunny-side up. Season with salt. Set aside.

5.For the plantains, fry plantain halves for 4 minutes or until golden.

6.To serve, put brown rice, a portion of the filling, 1 egg, and plantain half on plate.

Recipe #7 –Tofu Scramble

Ingredients:
- 2 tablespoons olive oil
- ½ onion, chopped
- 5 mushrooms, sliced
- 1 package firm tofu, crumbled
- 2 teaspoons curry powder
- Pinch of pepper
- Salsa, to taste
- 2 stalks green onion, chopped

Directions:

1. Heat olive oil in a nonstick skillet. Saute onions for 2 minutes or until translucent. Add in mushrooms. Cook for 4 minutes or until tender.

2. Place crumbled tofu into the mixture. Season with curry powder and pepper. Continue sautéing for 10 minutes.

3. Add in green onions and salsa. Scramble for 2 minutes. Serve.

Recipe #8 – Bulgur Wheat Salad With Orange Segments

Ingredients:
- 2 cups water
- 1 cup bulgur wheat
- 1 green pepper, diced
- ½ cucumber, diced
- 1 lemon rind, grated
- ½ cup fresh mint, chopped
- 4 tablespoons almonds, roasted
- 1 lemon, freshly squeezed
- 2 seedless oranges, cut into segments
- Pinch of salt
- Pinch of ground black pepper
- Fresh mint sprigs, to garnish

Directions:

1.Put together water and bulgur wheat in a bowl. Set aside for 20 minutes.

2.Drain soaked bulgur wheat using a colander. Squeeze out as much liquid. Transfer to a bowl.

3.Add green pepper, cucumber, lemon rind, mint, and toasted almonds. Put lemon juice. Mix well.

4.Add orange segments and juice into the bulgur mixture. Season with salt and pepper. Mix. Garnish with mint sprigs.

Recipe #9 – Carrot And Apple Shake

Ingredients:
- 1 cup crushed ice
- 1 carrot, chopped
- 1 apple, chopped
- ½ cup cold low-fat milk
- 1 tsp. stevia

Directions:
1. Put together crushed ice, chopped carrots and apples, milk, and stevia in a blender.
2. Blend until smooth and creamy.
3. Pour over glasses. Serve.

Recipe #10 - Fried Lady Fingers

Ingredients:
- 6 lady finger bananas, just ripe, halved lengthwise
- 2 Tbsp. coconut sugar
- coconut oil
- clarified butter

Directions:

1.Lightly grease a non-stick skillet with coconut oil.

2.Fry lady finger bananas for 4 minutes or until golden. Transfer to a plate.

3.Brush the tops of each banana with clarified butter. Sprinkle coconut sugar on top. Serve.

Recipe #11 - Dried Fruits Muesli

Ingredients:
Dry ingredients
•½ cup oat bran
•1 cup old-fashioned rolled oats
•½ tsp. nutmeg powder
•½ tsp. cinnamon powder
•½ cup dried apples, crushed
•¼ cup raisins
•½ cup dried peaches, crushed
•¼ cup pecan, roasted, store-bought, chopped
Wet ingredients
•6 pieces yogurt, divided
•1½ tsp. maple syrup, divided
Directions:
1.Combine oat bran, rolled oats, nutmeg powder, cinnamon powder, dried apples, raisins, peaches, and pecans in dry ingredients in a large bowl.
2.Pour half of the dry mixture into another bowl.
3.Add in maple syrup and 1 serving of yogurt.
4.Place inside the fridge to chill for 30 minutes. Serve.

Recipe #12 - Blueberry Pancakes

Ingredients:
- 3 tsp. baking powder
- 1 cup all-purpose flour
- ½ cup frozen blueberries, thawed
- 1 egg, whisked
- 2 Tbsp. pure maple syrup
- ⅛ tsp. salt
- ½ cup sour cream, low-fat
- 1 cup low-fat milk
- 2½ Tbsp. light olive oil
- 1 Tbsp. fresh blueberries, for garnish

Directions:
1. Using a blender, pour baking powder, all-purpose flour, blueberries, egg, sour cream, milk, maple syrup, salt, and olive oil. Process until the mixture is smooth.
2. Pour baking powder, all-purpose flour, frozen blueberries, egg, maple syrup, salt, sour cream, low fat milk, and olive oil into a plastic bottle with squeeze-tip. Seal and then shake well.
3. Meanwhile, heat a nonstick skillet. Pour just the right amount of batter, about ¼ cup into the heated skillet. Cook for 3 minutes or until the edges are set and the center is bubbling.
4. Flip pancakes to the other side and cook for another 2 minutes.
5. Transfer to a holding plate. Repeat the same cooking procedure for the remaining batter.

6.Garnish each pancake with blueberries. Serve.

Recipe #13 – Baked Omelet With Baby Spinach

Ingredients:
- 6 eggs, medium-sized, whisked until frothy
- 1 garlic clove, large, minced
- 1 white onion, minced
- 2 cups fresh baby spinach
- ¼ cup Parmesan cheese, shredded, divided
- 1 Tbsp. pumpkin seeds, shelled, roasted
- ½ Tbsp. olive oil

Directions:

1.Preheat the oven to 375 degrees F. lightly grease cups of muffin tins.

2.Meanwhile, in a skillet, heat the olive oil. Saute garlic and onion for 3 minutes or until limp and translucent. Add in baby spinach and bell peppers. Cook until spinach is wilted. Transfer to a holding plate.

3.Put together eggs and half of Parmesan cheese in a bowl.

4.Put just the right amount of stir-fried vegetables into the muffin cups.

5.Sprinkle pumpkin seeds on top. Pour egg mixture into the cup. Scatter parmesan cheese on top.

6.Place muffin tins into the oven. Bake for 25 minutes or until the eggs are set and the cheese turns golden brown.

7.Remove from the oven. Transfer to a wire rack and let cool for 5 minutes. Extract omelets from the muffin tins. Serve.

Chapter 2 – Dash Diet Lunch Menus

Recipe #14 - Curry Tuna Salad In Lettuce Wraps
Ingredients:

For the onion pickle

- •1 onion, sliced thinly
- •Pinch of sea salt

For the filling

- •1 Tbsp. tuna brine
- •1 can tuna chunks in water, drained
- •1 Tbsp. Greek yogurt
- •Dash of Spanish paprika
- •1 Tbsp. English mustard
- •Dash of curry powder
- •Pinch of sea salt
- •Pinch of white pepper
- •4 large Romaine lettuce leaves, chilled

Directions:

1.For the onion pickle, mash onion slices using your hands. Season with salt. Set aside, uncovered for 15 minutes.

2.Rinse onions under running water and make sure to drain well. Set aside.

3.For the tuna filling, put together tuna brine, tuna chunks Greek yogurt, Spanish paprika, English mustard, curry powder, salt, white pepper, and green chili in a large bowl. Place inside the fridge to chill for 1 hour or until ready to use.

4.To serve, spread just the right amount of filling along the inner spine of the lettuce leaf. Serve with the onion pickle on the side.

Recipe #15 - Grilled Tuna Fillets With Tomato Salad On The Side

Ingredients:
For the Tomato Salad
- 2 red salad tomatoes, ripe, cubed
- ¼ pound cherry tomatoes, quartered
- 2 beefsteak tomatoes, unripe, cubed
- 1 Tbsp. balsamic vinegar
- Pinch of sea salt
- Pinch of black pepper
- 1 leek, minced
- Pinch of fresh cilantro, minced

For the Fish fillets
- 4 tuna fillets, about ½-inch thick
- 2 Tbsp. Spanish paprika powder
- 1 lime, sliced into wedges
- 1 tsp. red pepper flakes
- ½ tsp. sea salt
- olive oil for brushing

Directions:
1. For the tomato salad, put together red salad tomatoes, cherry tomatoes, beefsteak tomatoes, balsamic vinegar, salt, pepper, leek and cilantro in a lidded, non-reactive container. Toss all ingredients until well-combined. Place inside the fridge to chill until ready to serve.

2.For the tuna grill, set the grill pan to medium heat. Lightly grease the grill surface with olive oil.

3.Put together red pepper flakes, Spanish paprika, and salt in a bowl. Use the mixture to rub all sides of the fish fillets. Grill for 5 minutes on one side. Flip to the other side and grill for 3 minutes.

4.Transfer to a holding plate. Cover fish with aluminum foil. Let sit for 5 minutes.

5.To serve, place one tuna fillet on a plate. Put just the right amount of tomato salad. Squeeze lime juice all over.

Recipe #16 - Asparagus Rice

Ingredients:
- 3 cups brown rice, cooked
- ½ pound asparagus, thick-stemmed, sliced into long slivers
- vegetable stock, low sodium
- Pinch of salt
- Pinch of black pepper
- ¼ cup fresh parsley, minced

Directions:

1. Put brown rice and asparagus into rice cooker. Pour vegetable stock. Season with salt and pepper. Secure the lid. Cook for 45 minutes to 1 hour.

2. Ladle just the right amount of asparagus rice into bowls. Serve with your favorite low sodium dish.

Recipe #17 - Cauliflower And Broccoli Bake

Ingredients:
- 1 cauliflower head, sliced into bite-sized florets
- 1 broccoli head, sliced into bite-sized florets
- 2 garlic cloves, grated
- 1 tsp. whole coriander seeds, crushed
- Pinch of black pepper
- olive oil for drizzling
- Pinch of sea salt

Directions:

1. Preheat the oven to 400°F. Line a roasting tin with aluminum foil.
2. Season cauliflower and broccoli florets, and garlic cloves with coriander seeds, salt and black pepper.
3. Drizzle in olive oil. Toss all ingredients until well-combined.
4. Place inside the oven and bake for 25 minutes.
5. Remove from heat. Serve.

Recipe #18 – Classic Caesar Salad

Ingredients:
For the Croutons
- 2 Tbsp. olive oil
- 4 pieces breadsticks, cubed
- 2 Tbsp. garlic flakes, crushed
- 1 cup roasted chicken, cubed

For the Dressing
- 4 egg yolks, whisked
- 4 Tbsp. cane vinegar
- 2 canned anchovies in oil, drained, minced
- water, only if needed
- Pinch of sea salt
- Pinch of black pepper
- ¼ cup sour cream
- ¼ cup Parmesan cheese, grated
- 2 pounds Romaine lettuce, torn into bite-sized pieces

Directions:
1. For the croutons, heat oil in a nonstick skillet. Fry bread cubes until toasted. Add in garlic flakes. Toss well.
2. Tip in cubed chicken into the mixture. Mix well. Set aside.
3. For the dressing, whisk egg yolks cane vinegar, anchovies, water, salt, pepper, sour cream, and Parmesan cheese in a bowl.
4. To serve, put croutons, lettuce, and chicken into the salad bowl. Drizzle in just the right amount of dressing. Put salad on the side.

Recipe #19 - Chicken Pastel

Ingredients:
- 1 cup sweet potato mash
- ¼ cup sour cream

For the Pie Filling
- 2 Tbsp. olive oil
- ½ cup white onion, minced
- 2 Tbsp. garlic, minced
- ¼ pound chicken thigh fillets, minced
- ¼ cup potatoes, diced
- ¼ cup frozen peas, thawed
- ¼ cup carrots, diced
- 1 can button mushrooms, pieces and stems
- ¼ cup chicken stock, unsalted
- Pinch of sea salt
- Pinch of white pepper

Directions:

1. Preheat the oven to 350 degrees °F.

2. For the pie filling, heat the olive oil in a Dutch oven. Saute onion and garlic for 3 minutes or until limp and translucent.

3. Add in chicken. Cook until the meat turns brown. Tip in potatoes, peas carrots, button mushrooms, and chicken stock into the Dutch oven. Season with salt and pepper. Stir well.

4. Bring mixture to a boil. Reduce the heat Allow to simmer fo 10 minutes or until most of liquid is reduced.

5.Turn off the heat. Add in sour cream. Adjust seasoning if needed.

6.For the pies: put just the right amount of filling into oven-safe ramekins. Put sweet potato mash on top.

7.Place ramekins on a baking sheet. Bake for 20 minutes. Allow to cool before serving.

Recipe #20 - Pan Fried Tilapia

Ingredients:
- 2 tilapia fillet
- 2 Tbsp. butter
- 1 Tbsp. fresh cilantro, minced, for garnish
- 2 tsp. Spanish paprika powder
- Pinch of sea salt
- olive oil for shallow frying

Directions:

1.Combine Spanish paprika powder and salt in a small bowl. Use this mixture to rub all over tilapia. Set aside to drain for 10 minutes in a colander.

2.Heat the olive oil into a nonstick skillet. Fry tilapia fillets until golden and crisp all over.

3.Place fillets on a plate. Garnish with fresh cilantro. Serve.

Recipe #21: Roasted Veggies Salad

Ingredients:
For the roasted carrots
•½ Tbsp. olive oil
•2 carrots, cubed
•2 tsp. cumin powder
•½ cup cashew nuts, raw, halved
•Pinch of sea salt
•Pinch of black pepper, to taste
For the lemon vinaigrette
•1 lemon, juiced
•1 tsp. extra virgin olive oil
•Pinch of sea salt
•Pinch of black pepper
•1 Tbsp. stevia
For the salad greens
•2 bags arugula, chopped
•2 bags baby spinach, chopped
Directions:
1.Preheat the oven to 400 degrees F. Line a baking sheet with parchment paper.
2.Put together olive oil, carrots, cumin powder, and cashew nuts in a bowl. Season with salt and pepper.
3.Place mixture onto the baking sheet. Roast for 30 minutes.
4.Remove from the oven and allow to cool for few minutes.

5.To make the lemon vinaigrette, combine lemon juice, olive oil, salt, pepper, and stevia in a separate bowl.
6.Drizzle in dressing over cooked carrots. Set aside.
7.Put together arugula, baby spinach, and roasted veggies in a salad bowl. Toss well to combine.
8.To serve drizzle in just the right amo8unt of vinaigrette over salad.

Chapter 3 – Dash Diet Dinner Recipes

Recipe #22 - Mackerel Steaks In Garlicky Buttery Sauce

Ingredients:
- 2 pieces Spanish mackerel steaks
- 2 Tbsp. olive oil
- 2 Tbsp. butter, divided
- ¼ cup garlic, grate
- Pinch of sea salt to taste

Directions:
1.Season Spanish mackerel steaks with just small amount of salt. Set aside.
2.Meanwhile heat the olive oil in a non-stick skillet. Saute garlic for 3 minutes or until golden. Set aside.
3.Add in half of the butter into the same skillet. Fry mackerel steaks for 4 minutes. Set aside.
4.Add in remaining butter. Cook fish thoroughly for 5 minutes. Garnish with garlic on top. Serve.

Recipe #23 - Garlicky Boodles

Ingredients:
- Broccoli noodles – also known as Boodles, spiralled into noodles using a spiralizer

For the broccoli
- 2 broccoli head, sliced into bite-sized florets
- 2 Tbsp. clarified butter
- 2 Tbsp. water
- Pinch of sea salt

For the Dressing
- 2 Tbsp. clarified butter
- 2 Tbsp. extra virgin olive oil
- 2 Tbsp. fried garlic flakes, crumbled
- 2 Tbsp. lemon juice, freshly-squeezed
- ¼ cup cashew nuts, chopped, toasted
- Pinch of sea salt
- Pinch of black pepper, to taste
- Dash of red pepper flakes

Directions:
1. For the broccoli noodles, layer them into the base of a microwave-safe dish.
2. Put the broccoli florets on top. Pour water and butter. Season with salt. Seal using saran wrap.
3. Microwave for 3 minutes. Remove from the oven. Remove saran wrap. Drain broccoli florets and broccoli noodles separately. Drain excess liquid.
4. To serve, put broccoli florets in a bowl. Season with clarified butter.

5.Place broccoli noodles in a bowl. In another bowl, combine olive oil, garlic flakes, lemon juice, cashew nuts, salt, pepper, and red pepper flakes. Mix well.
6.Pour dressing over the noodles. Top with broccoli florets. Serve.

Recipe #24 - Chicken And Mushrooms In Lettuce Wraps

Ingredients:
•6 iceberg lettuce leaves, chilled
For the filling
•1 Tbsp. olive oil
•2 fresh Portabella mushrooms, sliced thinly
•1 onion, minced
•1 garlic clove, minced
•¾ pound lean ground chicken
•1 tsp. ginger, grated
•1 carrot, julienned
•1 Tbsp. white vinegar
•1 Tbsp. catsup
•1 can chestnuts, minced
•1 tsp. sesame oil
Directions:

1.Pour olive oil into a non-stick skillet. Add in Portabella mushrooms. Cook for 3 minutes or until brown on both sides. Set aside.

2.In the same skillet, saute onion and garlic for 3 minutes or until fragrant and translucent. Stir in ground chicken. Cook for 4 minutes or until the meat is no

longer pink.

3.Stir in ginger, carrot, white vinegar, catsup, and chestnuts into the skillet. Cook for 5 minutes or until the sauce thickens. Remove from heat.

4.To serve, spoon equal amounts into lettuce leaves.

Recipe #25 - Mango Salad

Ingredients:
For the Dressing
- 1 tablespoons lime juice, freshly squeezed
- ⅛ teaspoon maple syrup
- Pinch of sea salt
- 1 mango, ripe, cubed
- 1 kiwi fruit, quartered
- ½ cup fresh blueberries
- 1 strawberry, quartered

Directions:

1. To make the dressing, pour lime juice, maple syrup, and salt into a bottle with tight fitting lid. Seal. Shake well.
2. Put mango, kiwi, blueberries, and strawberry into a large salad bowl. Drizzle in just the right amount of dressing. Toss well to combine. Serve.

Recipe #26 – Stir-Fried Cauliflower and Broccoli Florets

Ingredients:
- 2 garlic cloves, minced
- 1 onion, minced
- 1 red bell pepper, cubed
- 2 heads broccoli, sliced into bite-sized florets
- 2 heads cauliflower, sliced into bite-sized florets
- 2 tablespoons vegetable stock
- 1 tablespoons coconut oil
- Pinch of sea salt
- Pinch of white pepper

Directions:

1.Pour oil into wok set over medium heat. Add in and sauté garlic and shallot until limp and aromatic. Add in remaining ingredients.

2.Cook only until broccoli turns a shade brighter. This will allow veggies to remain crisp but tender. Turn off heat. Taste; season lightly.

3.Divide into equal portions. Serve.

Recipe #27 - Tuna Steaks With Cauliflower Pops

Ingredients:
For the cauliflower pops
- 1 cauliflower head, cut into bite-sized florets
- Dash of cayenne powder
- Pinch of white pepper
- 2 Tbsp. olive oil

For the tuna steaks
- 2 bone-in tuna steaks
- Pinch of sea salt
- 1 Tbsp. olive oil

For Garnish
- 2 Tbsp. toasted garlic flakes
- ½ lemon, cut into wedges

Directions:
1. Preheat the oven to 350 degrees F.
2. Toss cauliflower florets, cayenne powder, salt, and white pepper in a paper bag. Seal the bag and shake well. Make sure all the florets are well coated.
3. Put on the baking sheets. Drizzle in olive oil all over. Bake for 15 minutes.
4. Remove from the oven and allow to cool. Set aside.
5. Lightly season tuna steaks with salt.
6. Heat the oil in a nonstick skillet. Once its smoky and hot, slide tuna steaks. Fry for 3 minutes or until both sides are browned.
7. Transfer to a holding plate. Cover with aluminum foil and let sit for 5 minutes.

8.To serve, place steaks on plates. Sprinkle toasted garlic flakes on top. Serve with cauliflower pops on the side. Squeeze in lemon all over the dish.

Recipe #28 - Bell Pepper And Artichoke Pie

Ingredients:
For the Pie Filling
- 1 Tbsp. olive oil
- 1 garlic clove, minced
- ½ cup lean ground beef
- 1 green bell pepper, diced
- 1 red bell pepper, diced
- 1 artichoke hearts, diced
- 1/16 tsp. cumin powder
- Pinch of sea salt
- Pinch of white pepper

Directions:
1. Preheat the oven to 350 degrees F.
2. For the pie filling, heat the oil into a nonstick skillet. Saute the garlic for 3 minutes or until fragrant.
1. Stir in ground beef. Cook until the meat becomes brown and larger clumps are broken into small pieces.
2. Put green bell and red bell pepper artichoke hearts, cumin powder, salt, and pepper into the Dutch oven. Stir well. Adjust seasoning if needed.
3. For the pies, put just the right amount of pie filling into oven-safe ramekins.
4. Put ramekins on a baking sheet and bake for 20 minutes. Serve.

Recipe # 29 – Vegetarian Tacos

Ingredients:
- 3 tablespoons canned black beans
- 3 tablespoons canned corn kernels
- 3 tablespoons salsa
- 3 tablespoons cheddar cheese, shredded
- Olive oil
- ½ lb vegetarian sausage, crumbled
- 1 teaspoon lemon juice, freshly squeezed
- ¼ teaspoon chili powder
- 4 corn tortilla shells
- 2/3 cup lettuce, shredded

Directions:

1.Put together black beans, corn kernels, salsa, and cheddar cheese in a bowl. Mix well until all ingredients are well-combined.

2.Meanwhile, heat the olive oil in a skillet. Cook vegetarian sausage for 2 minutes. Squeeze in lemon juice and a bit of chili powder.

3.Divide cooked sausage mixture among tortilla shells. Put the bean-corn salsa. Top with shredded lettuce. Serve.

Recipe #30 - Veggie Noodles Salad With Chicken

Ingredients:
- 1 cup chicken, boiled, shredded
- ½ cup sour cream
- 1 package cream cheese
- 1 bird's eye chili, minced
- Pinch of sea salt
- Pinch of black pepper
- 1 Tbsp. extra virgin olive oil
- 1 zucchini, processed into flat ribbons using a spiralizer or vegetable peeler
- 2 cucumber, processed into flat ribbons using a spiralizer

Directions:

1. Put together shredded chicken, sour cream, cream cheese, bird's eye chili, salt, and pepper in a salad bowl. Adjust seasoning if needed.
2. Add in zucchini and cucumber ribbons. Toss well to combine Serve.

Recipe #31 - Fish Tacos With Tartar Sauce

Ingredients:
- 8 pieces wheat tortilla bread, warmed
- 2 lime, sliced into equal wedges

For the Fish
- 1½ pounds halibut fillets, sliced into slivers
- 2 eggs, whisked until frothy
- 1 cup panko breadcrumbs
- ½ cup all-purpose flour
- ½ tsp. sweet paprika powder
- ¼ tsp. cayenne pepper
- Pinch of black pepper
- Pinch of salt

For the Tartar Sauce
- 2 Tbsp. capers in brine
- 1 cup mayonnaise, reduced fat
- ¼ cup parsley, minced
- ½ cup cilantro, minced
- 2 Tbsp. lemon juice, freshly squeezed

For garnish
- Avocado slices
- Cabbage, shredded
- 1 tomato, sliced

Directions:

1.Season halibut fillet slivers with salt, black pepper, sweet paprika, and cayenne pepper. Set aside to drain in a colander for 15 minutes.

2.Meanwhile, in a bowl, combined flour, eggs, and panko breadcrumbs into three separate bowls.

3.Dredge halibut fillet into this order: flour first, egg, and then coat with breadcrumbs. Place on a baking sheet. Repeat the same procedure for the remaining fillets.

4.Heat the olive oil in a nonstick skillet. Once the oil is hot and smoky, slide breaded fillets. Deep fry until golden brown. Drain on paper towels.

5.For the tartar sauce, put together capers in brine, mayonnaise, parsley, cilantro, and lemon juice in a bowl.

6.To serve, place fish fillets into soft tacos. Add in cabbage, avocadoes, and tomatoes. Put a dollop of tartar sauce. Squeeze lime juice over. Serve.

Recipe #32 - Beef Stroganoff In Zucchini Pasta

Ingredients:
- 2 zucchini, cooked, processed into flat noodles using a spiralizer

For the stroganoff
- 1 Tbsp. olive oil
- 1 pound lean beef
- 1 garlic clove, minced
- 1 onion, minced
- 1 Tbsp. almond flour
- 1 cup beef stock, unsalted
- Pinch of sea salt
- Pinch of white pepper, to taste
- ½ cup sour cream

Directions:
1. Heat the olive oil in a skillet. Cook ground beef for 5 minutes or until the meat is brown all over and large clumps are broken down. Set aside.
2. In the same skillet, sauté garlic and onion for 3 minutes or until fragrant and tender. Add in almond flour. Pour beef stock. Season with salt and pepper. Adjust seasoning if needed.
3. Secure the lid and cook for 15 minutes. Turn off the heat. Stir in sour cream. Let residual heat cook the sour cream.
4. To serve, plate zucchini noodles. Top with beef stroganoff. Serve.

Recipe #33 - Baked Salmon Fillets With Kale Chips

Ingredients:
For the kale chips
•1 pound fresh kale leaves
•2 Tbsp. olive oil
• Pinch of coarse or sea salt
For the salmon fillets
•2 salmon fillets
•½ cup sour cream
•¼ cup Parmigiano cheese, grated
For garnish
•Dash of sweet paprika
•½ lemon, cut into wedges
Directions:
1.Preheat the oven to 350°F or 175°C.
2.Put the kale leaves on baking sheets. Season lightly with salt. Drizzle in olive oil all over. Bake for 10 minutes or until the leaves' edges are golden brown.
3.Remove from the oven and let cool for few minutes.
4.For the salmon fillets, put together sour cream and Parmigiano cheese in a bowl.
5.Place salmon fillets on the baking dish. Pour just the right amount of cheese on top of fillets. Bake for 20 minutes.
6.Remove from the oven. Cover with aluminum foil. Allow to rest for 5 minutes.

7.To serve, place fillet on a plate. Sprinkle a sweet paprika on top. Put kale chips on the side of the plate. Squeeze lemon juice on fillet. Serve.

Recipe #34 - Carrot And Potato Mash

Ingredients:
- 2 cups water
- 2 small pieces potatoes, cubed
- 3 large pieces carrots, cubed
- 2 Tbsp. salt
- ½ cup half-and-half
- 1¼ cups Parmigiano-Reggiano, grated
- 1/16 tsp. cumin powder
- 1 Tbsp. lemon juice, freshly squeezed
- 1/16 tsp. black pepper

Directions:
1. Pour water into a Dutch oven. Place potatoes and carrots. Season with salt. Bring to a boil.
2. Reduce the heat and allow to simmer for 20 minutes or until the vegetables are tender.
3. Turn off the heat. Drain water.
4. Pour half and half, Parmigiano-Reggiano, cumin powder, lemon juice, and black pepper into the Dutch oven.
5. Place cooked potatoes and carrots into the potato masher and process vegetables until creamy. Adjust seasoning if needed. Serve.

Recipe #35 - Apple Cinnamon Chicken Chops

Ingredients:

For the chicken chops

• 4 pieces chicken pieces either wing or breast part will do
• Pinch of Spanish paprika
• Pinch of salt
• Pinch of pepper
• 1 tsp. olive oil

For the apple cinnamon base

• 2 apples, sliced thinly
• 1 white onion, sliced thinly
• Pinch of cayenne powder
• 2 Tbsp. brown sugar
• 2 tsp. cinnamon powder
• 1 tsp. olive oil
• 1 tsp. butter
• ½ cup apple cider vinegar

Directions:

1. Season chicken pieces with Spanish paprika, salt, and pepper.
2. Heat the olive oil into a nonstick skillet. Fry seasoned chicken for 5 minutes on both sides until golden.
3. Transfer to a plate and cover with aluminum foil. Let sit for 3 minutes.
4. To make the cinnamon apple base, saute apples and onions for 3 minutes or until translucent.

5. Meanwhile, dissolve cinnamon, cayenne, and brown sugar in apple cider vinegar in a small bowl. Pour mixture into the pan.

6.Return chicken pieces into the pan. Spoon cinnamon apple base on top. Secure the lid and cook for another 10 minutes.

7.Put lid on, and lower heat setting to simmer. Let lamb chops cook for another 10 to 12 minutes.

8.To serve, place chicken in individual plates. Ladle apple cinnamon on top.

Recipes

Breakfast

Eggs With Cheese

Egg whites are better than eggs, and this DASH diet recipe allows you to combine both.

Ingredients:

1 egg

2 egg whites

2 tablespoons fat-free milk

1 ounce grated cheddar cheese, reduced fat

1 green onion, chopped

1/4 cup tomato, chopped

2 slices whole wheat bread

Mix the egg and egg whites in a bowl and add the milk. Scramble the mixture in a non-stick frying pan until the eggs cook.

Meanwhile, toast the bread. Spoon the scrambled egg mixture onto the toasted bread and top with the cheese until it melts. Add the onion and the tomato.

Chicken Breakfast Burrito

Breakfast is the most important meal of the day and if you like to maximize your healthy food intake in the morning, this recipe is for you. To save time, you can cook the chicken the night before and keep it in the fridge.

Ingredients:

4 ounces cooked skinless chicken

1 whole wheat tortilla

1 cup fresh spinach

1 pear, sliced

2 tablespoons fat-free salad dressing

Slice the chicken into small bite-sized pieces and arrange them on the tortilla. Cover the meat with spinach and arrange the pear slices on top.

Drizzle with your choice of salad dressing - look for one that is fat-free; low calorie and low in sodium.

Wrap the tortilla around all the ingredients until it's a snug burrito.

Wheat Bagel With Apple

There's no need to give up your morning bagel when you're following the DASH plan. This recipe packs in some protein as well as whole grains and fruit.

Ingredients:

1 whole wheat, whole grain bagel

1 apple, sliced

2 tablespoons natural peanut butter

Spread the peanut butter on each side of the bagel (make sure you use a brand that has no added salt) and layer the apple slices on top of the peanut butter.

Fruit And Nut Parfait

A perfect blend of crisp and crunch, you'll enjoy the creamy yogurt and the crunchy walnuts.

Ingredients:

1 cup melon

1 banana

1 cup mixed berries

1 /4 cup raisins

1/2 cup walnuts

2 cups fat free vanilla yogurt

Cut the melon into chunks that are about the same size as your berries and slice the banana. Mix in a large bowl with the raisins and the walnuts.

Top with the yogurt and blend to combine. Chill for about 30 minutes and serve in two separate bowls.

Mango Smoothie

If you don't have a big appetite in the morning but you know you need to eat, try this smoothie.

Ingredients:

1 cup frozen or fresh mango

1 medium banana

1/4 cup fat-free yogurt, plain

1/2 cup fat-free milk

1 cup kale

1/4 cup whole oats

1 cup ice

Place the milk, yogurt and oats in a blender and combine on low speed for 30 seconds.

Add the mango, banana, kale and ice and blend on high speed until smooth and combined. You can eliminate the ice if you don't want a smoothie that tastes too frozen.

This makes one smoothie and it's great for sticking with the DASH plan when you need to dash out the door in the mornings.

Grapefruit Yogurt Bowl

Get creative and put a new spin on your favorite fruit salad.

Ingredients:

1/2 grapefruit

1 cup strawberries, chopped

1 teaspoon brown sugar

1 cup fat-free vanilla yogurt

1/4 cup walnuts

1/4 cup blueberries

Scoop out the grapefruit segments from the rind and place in a bowl. Add the strawberries and blueberries and combine. Toss the fruit mixture with the brown sugar.

Place the yogurt in the hollow grapefruit shell. Spoon the fruit mixture onto the yogurt and sprinkle the top with walnuts.

Rice Pilaf

This rice dish is inspired by South Asian pilau, which often include fruit and nuts, so it`s great for breakfast.

Ingredients:

2 1/4 cups vegetable stock

1 1/4 cups long grain brown rice

1/4 cup pistachios

1/4 cup dried apricots

3 tablespoons orange juice

1 1/2 tablespoons canola, coconut or sunflower oil

1/4 teaspoon saffron salt substitute to taste

Combine the rice, stock and saffron in a medium saucepan. Bring to a boil over high heat. Reduce the heat to low and cover, simmering until the rice has become tender and absorbed all the liquid. Transfer to a large bowl.

Combine the orange juice, oil and salt substitute in a small bowl. Pour this mixture over the rice.

Chop the apricots.

Heat a small skillet to medium and add the fruit and nuts, stirring continuously until the pistachios brown slightly and develop an oily appearance.

Toss the fruit and nuts with the flavored rice to mix.

Serve right away.

Homemade Granola

This homemade granola recipe is nutritionally dense and concentrates on healthy fats and natural, relatively unrefined sources of sugar.

Ingredients:

3 cups old-fashioned rolled oats

1 cup sliced almonds

1 cup raisins or dried cranberries

4 tablespoons flax seed

1/4 cup raw sugar

1/4 cup honey

1/4 cup sunflower or canola oil

1/2 teaspoon vanilla extract

1/2 teaspoon ground sugar

1/2 teaspoon allspice

1/2 teaspoon ground ginger

Combine the oats, almonds, flax, spices and sugar in a large bowl, mixing thoroughly.

In a separate bowl combine the honey, oil and vanilla extract. Pour the wet ingredient mixture into the dry ingredients, mixing with a spatula as you pour. Stir until the dry mixture is wet throughout.

Lightly grease one to two cookie sheets with sunflower oil or another monounsaturated fat. Pour the wet granola into the pans, patting it into place if necessary.

Bake in a 250 degree Fahrenheit oven for 90 minutes or until dry and lightly browned, stirring every 15 minutes. Break up chunks of granola as you stir to create the appropriate consistency.

Allow the mixture to cool, then combine with the dried fruit and store in an air-tight container.

Breakfast Sandwich

If you love eggs for breakfast, this recipe will help you enjoy them without the heart risk associated with large amounts of egg yolk. Flavorful mustard and tomatoes keep the open-faced sandwich interesting, so you won't miss the fat.

Ingredients:

2 egg whites

1/2 cup fresh spinach leaves

1 slice whole grain bread

1 small tomato

1 1/2 teaspoons olive oil

1 teaspoon prepared brown mustard

1/2 ounce slice reduced-fat cheddar cheese

Black pepper and paprika to taste

In a small pan, heat the olive oil to medium-high. Beat the egg whites and add to the hot oil, scrambling them until completely solid. Add the spinach and heat until wilted.

Spread the mustard onto the bread and place it on an oven-safe plate or baking sheet. Arrange tomato slices on top of the mustard, then top with the egg mixture and thinly-sliced cheddar cheese. Sprinkle with black pepper and sharp paprika to taste.

Bake in an oven or toaster oven at 400 degrees Fahrenheit until the bread is crisp and the cheese is melted and slightly browned.

Almond-Banana Toast

Putting the finished product under the broiler caramelizes the natural sugars in the banana, producing a delicious, gooey result that you'll also enjoy as a snack.

Ingredients:

2 slices whole grain bread

2 tablespoons smooth almond butter

1 small banana

ground cinnamon and nutmeg to taste

Toast the bread and arrange it on an oven-safe plate or a small baking sheet. Spread each slice with 1 tablespoon of almond butter.

Slice the banana into rounds of medium thickness and arrange them on top of the almond butter.

Sprinkle the surface with cinnamon and nutmeg, then place under the broiler for 2 to 3 minutes, or until the almond butter melts slightly and the bananas begin to brown.

Allow to cool and eat with your fingers, or dig in right away with a fork.

Lunch

Brown Rice And Beans

If you like Caribbean food, this is a must for you, and even if you don't, please give it a try.
Ingredients:
1 cup dark brown rice
2 cups water
1 teaspoon salt
3 tablespoons fresh orange juice
1 tablespoon olive oil
1/4 cup pine nuts
1 cup black beans, no salt added
3 stems fresh cilantro

Combine rice, water, salt, olive oil in a saucepan and simmer for about 45 minutes, until rice cooks.
Remove from heat and add pine nuts and orange juice. Stir in the black beans until combined. Top with fresh cilantro.
This recipe serves 6.

Tantalizing Tuna Melt

This is easy-to-make lunch recipe. Plus, you can pack it for take away!

Ingredients:
4 whole wheat flour tortillas
2 cans of chunk light tuna in water, drained
8 tomato slices
1/4 cup red onion, chopped
1/4 cup celery, chopped
2 tablespoons lemon juice
2 tablespoons extra virgin olive oil
2 slices low-fat mozzarella cheese
Ground black pepper

Empty the tuna out of the cans into a small bowl. Use a fork to mix it with the olive oil and lemon juice.
Add the celery and the onion. Sprinkle pepper into the mixture.
Preheat your oven to 325 degrees. Lay the tortillas on a cookie sheet and spoon the tuna mixture onto each one, dividing it evenly. Top each with two thick tomato slices and then cover with cheese.
Bake for about 10 minutes, until the cheese is melted. Remove from oven and let cool for 2 minutes. Roll the tortilla into a wrap and enjoy.
This recipe makes four tuna melts.

Pear And Walnut Salad

Not your usual salad but the combination of pear and walnut gives so much pleasure and a wonderful sweet-salty taste.
Ingredients:
6 cups of mixed lettuces and greens

3 pears, thinly sliced
1/4 cup toasted walnuts, chopped
1 fennel bulb, thinly sliced
2 tablespoons grated pecorino cheese
3 tablespoons extra virgin olive oil
3 tablespoons balsamic vinegar
Ground black pepper

Wash the lettuces and place in a large bowl. Spread the fennel and the pear over the lettuces and top with the cheese, oil, vinegar and pepper. Finish with the chopped walnuts.
This recipe serves 4 people.

Pasta Primavera

Pasta Primavera means pasta with fresh vegetables, so you always use the fresh vegetables of the season.
Ingredients:
12 ounces whole wheat pasta
1 garlic clove, chopped
1 red bell pepper, chopped
1 green bell pepper, chopped
1 yellow bell pepper, chopped
1 cucumber, chopped
1 red onion, chopped
1 can diced tomatoes, no salt added
2 tablespoons extra virgin olive oil
1 tablespoon lemon juice
1/2 teaspoon basil
1/2 teaspoon oregano

1/2 teaspoon rosemary
1/2 teaspoon parsley

Cook the pasta and drain. Rinse with cool water and shake in a strainer until excess water is removed. Pour into a large bowl. Add olive oil and lemon juice, toss pasta to coat.
Add the chopped vegetables and combine. Sprinkle with herbs and pour the can of tomatoes on the top, juices included.
Allow the salad to chill in the refrigerator for at least one hour. Serve alone or on top of large lettuce leaves. This recipe provides four generous servings.

Chicken Chili

Not your usual chili, I admit. (I mean, chicken in a chili?!) But thanks to the slow cooking process and the different veggies and spices, you won't notice a difference.
Ingredients:
10 ounces skinless chicken, cooked
28 ounces canned crushed tomatoes, no salt added
2 cups black beans, no salt added
1 red onion, diced
2 stalks of celery, diced
1 red bell pepper, diced
2 jalapeno peppers, diced
2 cloves of garlic, minced
2 tablespoons red pepper flakes
1 tablespoon black pepper

1 tablespoon oregano
1 tablespoon olive oil
1/4 cup water

In a large soup pot, cook the celery, onion, peppers and garlic in the olive oil for 5 minutes.
Add all remaining ingredients and cook, covered for 2 hours. Stir occasionally while it simmers.
This recipe makes 8 servings.

Citrus Shrimp Salad

Here is a simple gourmet salad recipe with an orange twist.
Ingredients:
1/2 pound cooked small salad shrimp, peeled and rinsed
1/4 cup freshly squeezed orange juice
1 tablespoon balsamic vinegar
6 cups spinach and lettuce mix
1 cucumber, chopped
2 oranges, peeled and chopped

Combine the shrimp with the orange juice, vinegar and cucumber and toss. Chill the mixture in the refrigerator for at least 30 minutes.
Place the mixture on top of the lettuce and spinach and sprinkle with orange segments.
This recipe provides 4 salad servings.

Turkey Salad Sandwich

A healthy DASH version of one of the most popular sandwich choices in the world.

Ingredients:

2 slices whole grain bread

1/2 cup shredded turkey

1 tablespoon fat free mayonnaise

1/4 cup chopped celery

1/4 cup chopped apple

1 large lettuce leaf

2 tomato slices

Ground black pepper

Mix the shredded turkey in a bowl with mayonnaise, celery, apple and ground pepper.

Lay the lettuce leaf on top of one bread piece. Scoop the turkey out of the bowl and onto the lettuce leaf. Top with the tomato slices and place the other piece of bread on top.

This recipe creates one turkey sandwich.

Carrot Curry

This smooth curry contains plenty of exciting spices, along with protein-rich low fat yogurt and bright, tangy cilantro. For a spicier version, substitute cayenne or Thai peppers for the jalapeno.

Ingredients:

5 cups low-sodium vegetable stock

1 pound carrots

164

1 large yellow onion

1 jalapeno pepper

1/4 cup cilantro leaves

1/4 cup low fat unsweetened yogurt

2 tablespoons lime or lemon juice

1 tablespoon sunflower oil

1 tablespoon fresh ginger

2 cloves garlic

2 teaspoons Madras curry powder

1 teaspoon black mustard seeds salt substitute to taste

Heat the olive oil in a large saucepan to medium.

Mince the garlic and ginger and chop the onion finely.

Add the mustard seed to the oil and allow it to pop, then add the ginger, garlic and onion. Cook for about 5 minutes, stirring continuously, or until the onions become translucent but not brown.

Remove the stem, seeds and ribs of the jalapeno and chop it finely, then add to the pan along with the curry powder.

Chop the carrots roughly and sauté with the other ingredients for about 3 minutes, or until the seasonings begin to toast. Pour in about half of the stock and bring the whole pot to a boil over high heat. Reduce to medium-low and simmer for about 5 minutes, or until the carrots become tender.

Remove the soup from the pot and place it in a blender or food processor. Process until the liquid is smooth, in batches if necessary, and return to the pan. Stir in the remaining stock and reheat.

Add yogurt, cilantro and lime juice, as well as salt substitute to taste. Garnish with additional cilantro and limes before serving.

Edamame Salad

Fresh, steamed soybeans are known as Edamame in Japan, and are eaten as an appetizer or part of other dishes. When served cold, these beans also make a great salad ingredient.

Ingredients:

1/2 pound fresh Edamame

1 pint cherry or grape tomatoes

1/4 cup red wine vinegar

1 1/2 tablespoons extra virgin olive oil

1 scallion

1 small bunch fresh dill weed

1 small bunch fresh mint

1/4 teaspoon black pepper

Place the soybeans in a steamer over about an inch of water. Cover and steam for approximately 5 minutes, or until the pods are bright green and the beans are crisp-tender. Rinse with cold water and remove from the pods.

Set the beans aside in a medium bowl and refrigerate.

Chop the mint and dill finely. Slice the green onion. Cut large cherry tomatoes into halves, leaving small ones whole.

Combine tomatoes, green onion, mint and dill in a medium bowl.

Mix oil, vinegar and black pepper in a small bowl and pour over the salad.

Serve chilled.

Dash Pasta Sauce

The DASH diet works best when you reduce the amount of meat in your diet, but many people don't know where to start. This vegetable-based pasta sauce proves that you don't need to have sausage or beef to make a meal special. Serve it with your favorite whole grain pasta.

Ingredients:

8 ounces canned low-sodium tomato sauce

6 ounces canned low-sodium tomato paste

2 medium zucchini

2 medium fresh tomatoes

2 small onions

3 cloves garlic

2 tablespoons olive oil

1 tablespoon dried oregano

1 tablespoon dried basil

1 teaspoon dried rosemary

1 cup water

Heat the olive oil in a medium-sized skillet.

Mince the garlic and onions. Chop the zucchini and tomatoes coarsely.

Add all vegetables to the pan and sauté for about 5 minutes over medium-high heat, or until the onions become slightly translucent.

Mix the tomato paste and water in a medium bowl until smooth. Add to the pan, along with the tomato sauce and herbs. Cover and reduce the heat to low. Simmer for 45 minutes or until the sauce reaches the desired consistency.

Season with salt substitute if desired.

Dinner

Salmon Salad

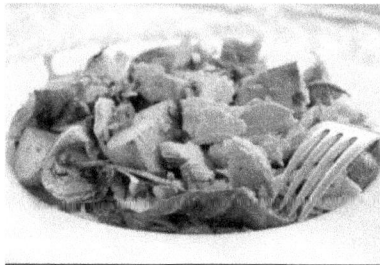

A quick and easy dinner recipe which has amazing anti-inflammatory effects, especially if you use wild salmon.
Ingredients:
4 salmon filets, 6 ounces each
2 tablespoons lemon juice
1 garlic clove, minced
8 lemon slices
2 tablespoons fresh Italian parsley
ground black pepper
6 cups mixed lettuce greens

2 tomatoes, chopped
1/4 cup toasted almonds, salt-free
1/4 cup extra virgin olive oil

Preheat the oven to 350 degrees. Cover the salmon
with lemon juice, garlic and lemon slices. Sprinkle with
parsley and pepper and cook for 15 minutes.
Mix the salad with lettuce, tomatoes, almonds and
olive oil. Place the salmon on top.
This recipe serves 4.

Chicken Kebab

This Middle East inspired recipe is perfect for the BBQ in summer.

Ingredients:

12 ounces cooked chicken, cut into pieces

2 red bell peppers, chopped

1 red onion, chopped

2 cups cherry or grape tomatoes

1 cup button mushrooms

1 cup pineapple chunks

2 tablespoons olive oil

Ground black pepper

Heat a grill or a grill pan and place the meat, vegetables and pineapple chunks on skewers in any pattern that appeals to you.

Brush each kebab with olive oil and sprinkle with pepper. Heat the kebabs on the grill, turning to ensure all sides are cooked. Remove from the grill and serve with a side of salad or a bowl of fruit.

This recipe serves 4 people (2 kebabs each).

Turkey Burgers

Okay, it's actually not a burger per se but once you have tasted it, you will never ever again look for the big yellow M signs by the road.

Ingredients:

1 pound ground turkey breast
1/3 cup whole grain oats
4 slices whole grain wheat bread
4 slices low fat cheddar cheese
1 cup raw spinach leaves
1 tomato, sliced
1/4 red onion, sliced into rings
Ground black pepper
1/4 cup chopped yellow onion
1/4 cup chopped red pepper
2 tablespoons fat free mayonnaise

Put the red pepper and yellow onion in a food processor and pulse until very fine. Combine with the turkey breast and the whole oats.

Heat a grill or a grill pan. While the grill heats up, form the turkey mixture into 4 patties of equal size. Grill on each side, until cooked and allow the cheese to melt before you remove from grill.

While they are cooking, toast the bread. Spread a light layer of mayonnaise on the bread and place one turkey patty on each slice. Top with spinach, tomato and red onion. Sprinkle with black pepper.

This makes four turkey burgers.

Bbq Chops

Barbecued pork may sound unhealthy and decadent, but you can substitute other meats to make your favorite pork recipes compatible with the DASH diet. This recipe uses "chops" of boneless chicken thighs, since the dark meat provides similar flavor intensity to that of lean pork. Add a fresh salad and this dish is ready to make a complete meal!

Ingredients:

1 1/2 pounds boneless chicken thighs

10 ounces low sodium condensed tomato soup

3 tablespoons red wine vinegar

2 tablespoons low sodium

Worcestershire sauce

1 small onion

3/4 cup water

1 teaspoon sharp paprika

1 teaspoon chili powder

1/4 teaspoon cinnamon

1/4 teaspoon black pepper

1/8 teaspoon cloves

Trim all fat from the chicken, cube, and set aside.

Combine all other ingredients in a large bowl, then transfer to a large skillet with high sides.

Heat to medium and add the chicken cubes, simmering for 30 minutes or until cooked thoroughly.

Serve with bread or 2/3 cup of brown rice.

Blackened Beef

Thinly sliced lean top round beef seared with strong spices makes for an exciting and flavorful main dish, especially when you pair it with stewed potatoes, onions and carrots

Ingredients:

1 pound lean top round of beef

6 medium red potatoes

4 large onions

3 large carrots

2 cups low-sodium beef broth

2 cups water

2 cloves garlic

1 bunch kale

2 tablespoons sharp paprika

1 tablespoon dried oregano

1 teaspoon chili powder

1 teaspoon powdered garlic

1/2 teaspoon black pepper

1/4 teaspoon red pepper

1/4 teaspoon mustard powder

Place the beef in the freezer until partially frozen.

Cut the potatoes into quarters, mince the garlic cloves, slice the carrots into rounds and remove the stems from the kale.

Chop the onions very finely to yield about 4 cups.

Combine paprika, oregano, garlic powder, chili powder, red and black peppers and dry mustard in a small bowl with a lid. Set aside.

Remove beef from freezer and slice it across the grain in strips about 1/8 inch thick. Sprinkle with the seasoning mix, covering all available surfaces.

Lightly grease a large heavy skillet or stockpot then preheat over high. Add the meat strips and sear, stirring continuously, for about 5 minutes.

Add the broth and water to the pan to deglaze, then add potatoes and garlic to the skillet. Allow the blackened spices to float to the top.

Cover and lower heat to medium, cooking for about 20 minutes or until potatoes are tender.

Add the carrots and place the kale on top of the dish. Cover and cook for an additional 10 minutes.

This dish can be served right from the skillet or pot.

Greek Pizza

Many DASH dieters find that they miss conventional pizza after they start their new healthier way of eating. Once you learn to make these pizzas at home, you won't miss delivery.

Ingredients:

10 ounces fresh or frozen spinach

3 1/4 cups low sodium marinara sauce

1 1/4 cups reduced-fat ricotta cheese

1 1/4 cups fresh mint

1 cup fresh fennel

1 whole grain 14 inch pizza crust or equivalent dough

3/4 cup feta cheese crumbles

4 plum tomatoes

1 teaspoon strongly-flavored olive oil

1 teaspoon cornmeal

salt substitute and black pepper to taste

Heat a pizza stone or cookie sheet in the oven at 500 degrees Fahrenheit. Sprinkle a pizza peel with cornmeal to prevent sticking. If you are using a pizza crust, follow package instructions to prepare it for topping.

Chop the mint, tomatoes, fennel and spinach.

Heat the olive oil in a large skillet to medium-high.

Add the chopped fennel and sauté for five minutes, or until slightly translucent. Reduce the heat to medium-low.

Drain all water from the spinach and add it to the fennel. Season with black pepper and salt substitute according to your preferences.

Place the raw dough on the pizza peel and transfer it to the baking stone or sheet.

Cook for 5 minutes at 500 degrees and remove from oven.

Spread the sauce over the pizza crust, then top with the spinach and fennel mixture. Spoon the ricotta in small quantities over the vegetable mixture, but do not try to spread it.

Add feta crumbles and bake for another 15 minutes, or until the crust is cooked completely and the edges are lightly browned.

Combine the mint and tomatoes in a separate bowl, then sprinkle them over the surface of the pizza before cutting.

Lentil Chili

This tasty vegetarian alternative to conventional chili is hearty and flavorful, with bulgur wheat and lentils replacing the usual fatty beef and chili beans.

Ingredients:

3 cups low-sodium vegetable broth

2 cups or one can chopped tomatoes

1 cup bulgur wheat

1 cup dried lentils

1 medium white onion

4 cloves garlic

2 tablespoons canola oil

2 1/2 tablespoons chili powder

1 tablespoon cumin powder

1/2 teaspoon cinnamon

Salt substitute and pepper to taste

Heat the oil to medium-high in a large pot.

Mince the onion and garlic, then add them to the pot and cook for 5 minutes, stirring continuously. When the alliums have become slightly translucent, add the wheat and lentils, followed by the broth.

Stir to combine, then add the tomatoes and spices.

Bring to a boil over high heat, then reduce to low and cover. Simmer for 30 minutes or until the lentils just begin to fall apart.

Add salt substitute and pepper to taste and serve hot.

Grilled Chicken

This basic chicken dish is easy to make on any outdoor grill. You won't miss the extra fat!

Ingredients:

4 bone-in chicken breasts with skin

2 cloves garlic

salt-free herb seasoning mix

Heat a gas or charcoal grill to medium heat.

Fold non-stick aluminum foil into a boat shape for each chicken breast.

Cut the garlic cloves in half and rub the cut surfaces over the skin of the chicken breasts. Sprinkle with seasoning mix to taste and place the chicken breasts in the boats, skin side down.

Grill for 45 minutes or until the center reaches 160 degrees Fahrenheit, turning the chicken once every 10 to 15 minutes.

Asian Cod

This spicy Asian fish recipe provides plenty of healthy polyunsaturated omega-3 fatty acids, along with the rich flavors of miso and chili paste. If cod is unavailable, use any firm, flaky white fish that can be cut into thick steaks.

Ingredients:

1 pound cod

3 tablespoons low-salt sweet white miso

1 tablespoon garlic-chili paste

2 tablespoons apple juice

2 tablespoons unprocessed cane sugar, such as turbinado

Mix together all raw ingredients except for the fish.

Take a piece of plastic wrap and spread it over the counter or a cutting board, then apply a layer of miso marinade a little larger than the total surface area of the fish.

Place a piece of cheesecloth on top of the marinade layer. Wrap the cheesecloth around the fish, then apply marinade to the top side. Wrap the plastic around the fish and its wrapping, then place the plastic bundle into a freezer bag.

Place in the refrigerator for two hours to overnight.

Remove the fish from the refrigerator and peel away the plastic and cheesecloth layers.

Heat a large nonstick frying pan over medium heat and place the fish in it. Cook on both sides until the fish is opaque and flaky throughout.

Serve with low-sodium miso soup, rice and Japanese pickles.

Discard any unused marinade for safety reasons.

Chinese Beef

This dish uses thinly-sliced lean beef, heart-friendly oils and fresh ginger to recreate a classic Chinese restaurant favorite.

Ingredients:

3/4 pound thinly-sliced flank or sirloin steak

1 medium onion

1 pound mushrooms

1 pound broccoli

2 tablespoons peanut oil

1 tablespoon rice vinegar

1 tablespoon fresh ginger

3 cloves fresh garlic

red pepper flakes to taste

salt substitute to taste

In a deep skillet or wok, heat 1 tablespoon of peanut oil on high.

Mince the ginger and onion and add to the hot pan, frying for about a minute.

Season with salt substitute to taste.

Crush the garlic, slice the mushrooms and chop the broccoli. Add 1 teaspoon of garlic and the mushrooms to the pan.

Cook for about 2 minutes, stirring throughout, or until the mushrooms soften and the onions become translucent.

Add the broccoli and cook for about 3 minutes or until it is bright green and still slightly crisp.

Remove the vegetables to a bowl.

Add the remaining tablespoon of peanut oil to the pan and allow it to heat.

Add the beef strips and the remaining garlic, cooking for about 2 minutes. Sprinkle in the vinegar and red pepper flakes, followed by the vegetables. Stir to combine and remove from the heat immediately.

Serve over short grain brown rice.

Conclusion

Thanks again for downloading this book.
I hope this book has helped you find different kinds of healthy and nutritious recipes and variations for breakfast, lunch, and dinner meals.
The next step is to create a weekly meal plan by using all the recipes found here. When it comes to following a specific diet, it is vital that you plan ahead so that you will not end up overeating again.

www.ingramcontent.com/pod-product-compliance
Lightning Source LLC
Chambersburg PA
CBHW062136020426
42335CB00013B/1231